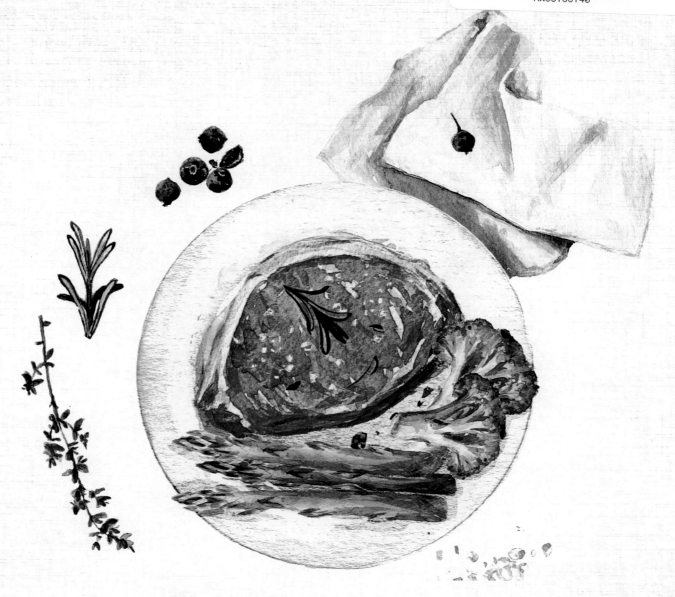

Make it Fast, Cook it Slow

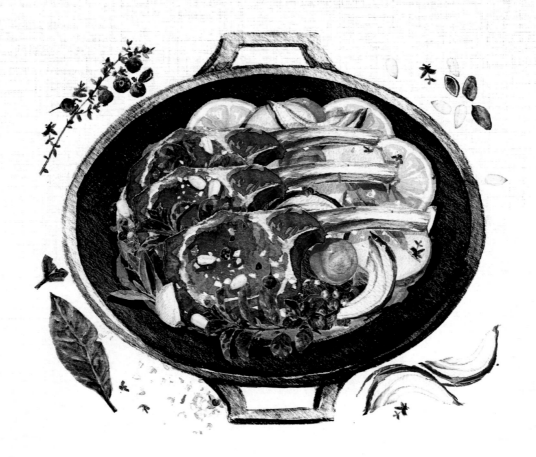

If a dream of yours is to create delicious and nourishing meals every night of the week, but you simply do not have time, I am here to share easy one pot wonder recipes with you to make that desire come true.

You no longer have to slave in the kitchen to create an amazing dish and the best part is that you can create healthy recipes every night of the week without having numerous dishes to wash! These recipes are also low carb, making them an excellent addition to a ketogenic diet.

One pot recipes only require one pot or one dish and take very minimal prep time on your end! A one pot wonder means that you can whip out your slow cooker, roasting pan or skillet and get cooking without the fuss. Not only are one pot wonders easy to make, they are also incredibly nourishing. Your body has the ability to absorb all of the wonderful vitamins and minerals from each ingredient since they all cook together in one pot.

If you want to eat healthy every night, without any hassle, this will become your new go-to book.

Introduction

Slow Cooker Recipes
Soups

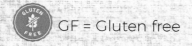 GF = Gluten free   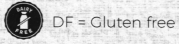 DF = Gluten free   V = Vegetarian

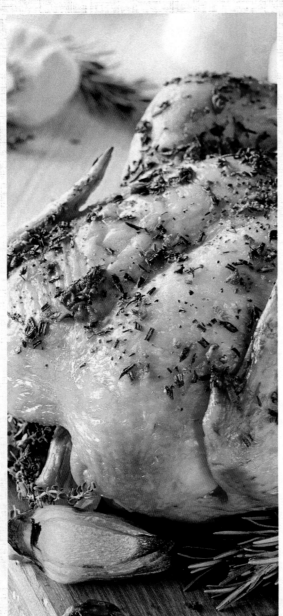

Stews

Garlicky Beef Stew (GF, DF) **23**

Creamy Mushroom Beef Stew (GF) **24**

Cinnamon Butternut Beef Stew (GF, DF) **25**

Hamburger Stew (GF) **26**

Fire Roasted Vegetable Stew (GF, DF, V) **27**

Hot Pepper Chicken Stew (GF, DF) **28**

Slow Cooked Meats

Rosemary Peppered Steak (GF, DF) **30**

BBQ Sirloin Steak (GF) **31**

Creamy Chicken & Sausage (GF) **32**

Italian Beef (GF, DF) **33**

Zesty Meatballs (GF, DF) **34**

Lemon & Herb Whole Chicken (GF, DF) **35**

Italian Chicken Parmesan (GF) **36**

Peanut Curried Chicken (GF, DF) **37**

Chicken Teriyaki (GF, DF) **38**

Peppercorn & Sage Pork Loin (GF) **39**

Thousand Island Pork Loin (GF, DF) **40**

Hickory Baby Back Ribs (GF) **41**

Other Slow Cooked Favorites

Southwest Tacos With Coconut Tortillas (GF, DF) **43**

Stuffed Collard Greens (GF, DF) **44**

Wild Dill Salmon (GF, DF) **45**

Pizza Chicken (GF) **46**

Chicken Stuffed Peppers (GF, DF) **47**

 GF = Gluten free   DF = Gluten free   V = Vegetarian

4

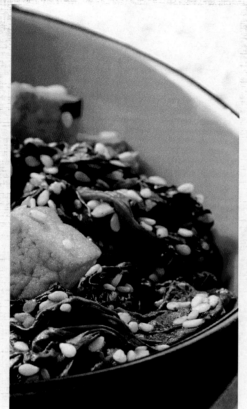

Skillet Recipes

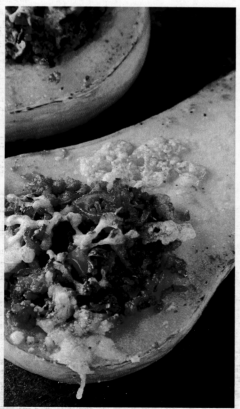

Roasting Pan Recipes

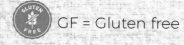 GF = Gluten free   DF = Gluten free   V = Vegetarian

Different One Pot
COOKING METHODS

One of the great things about one pot cooking is that there are a number of different methods you can use. You are not limited to only using a slow cooker or a roasting pan. In this book, I share recipes for slow cookers, skillets and roasting pans so that you never get tired of the same old cooking method. Here are some of the benefits of using each of these one pot cooking methods.

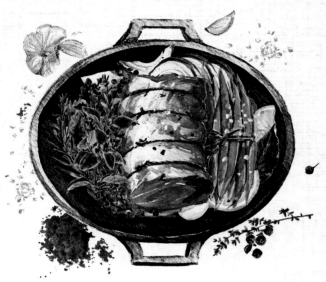

Slow Cooker:
The slow cooker is one of the most traditionally used one pot cooking methods. You truly can't get much easier than tossing the ingredients into the base of the cooker, turning it on and leaving it to cook for the day. Slow cookers are excellent for people living busy lives who want a home-cooked meal ready and hot for when they come home from a long day or night.

Skillet:
Skillet recipes are also super convenient. While you have to do more active work than if you were using a slow cooker, the skillet is great because you have very minimal dish washing to do once your meal is cooked! Simply add the ingredients to the pan and cook away.

Roasting Pan:
A roasting pan is traditionally used for cooking things like turkey and chicken, but you can do so much more! You can make things like roasted vegetables and even a roasted leg of lamb. It takes very little work on your end and all you need to do is prep the ingredients, place them in the pan and cook them in the oven.

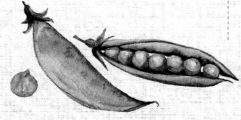

Benefits
OF ONE POT COOKING

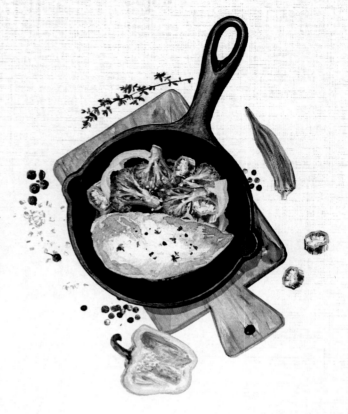

Besides the fact that one pot cooking is super easy and takes very little prep and clean-up work on your end, there are even more benefits you will want to know about! Here are some of the benefits one pot cooking holds:

•Useful Year Round:
Although many of us may think about the one pot cooking method being used in the colder months when we crave a hot meal, one pot cooking is really great for all-year-round cooking. The benefit of one pot cooking in the summer is that if you use a slow cooker, you don't have to worry about turning your oven on and heating up your house!.

• Time-Saver:
We all know that time is short nowadays and not everyone has time to make a home cooked meal every night. With one pot cooking, now you can achieve this with very minimal effort.

•Nutritious:
By using the one pot cooking method, you can toss in as many fiber-rich veggies as you would like and cook them all together without having to wash a ton of dishes. No more excuses for skimping on your veggies!

•Transportable:
Cooking for friends and family? If you decide to cook your meal in a slow cooker, you can easily transport it to your next dinner party.

As you can see, there is more than one reason to consider one pot cooking: not only do you pack in a healthy dose of nutritional value in each meal, you get to enjoy a delicious meal that hits the spot every day.

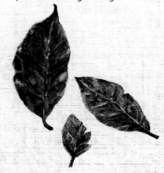

Tips
On Making A Delicious One Pot Wonder

One pot cooking is by no means rocket science, but there are some tricks to make it the best dish possible! Through experience, I have a few tricks up my sleeve that I would like to share with you. Here are some tips to make your one pot wonder even more delicious:

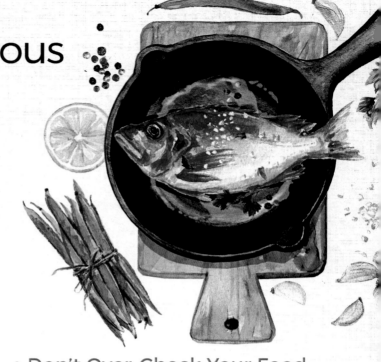

• Use Seasoning:
Don't be afraid to use seasoning. Get creative and try different flavors to bring the most out of your dish.

• Go Easy on the Liquid:
When it comes to slow cookers, you don't necessarily always need to use a ton of liquid. Since your slow cooker has a tight lid, the liquid isn't going to evaporate as it would in a stock pot. The liquid you use should only just cover the meat and veggies you have at the base of the cooker.

• Use the Low Setting When Possible:
When using a slow cooker, you will want to use the low setting when possible. Gently heating brings out the flavors more than always cooking your foods on high and it can also help to hold onto the nutritional value a little bit more.

• Don't Over-Check Your Food:
Checking to see how your food is coming along once, whether that be in the slow cooker or the oven, is normally okay, but over-checking is not. By opening the lid or opening the door of the oven, you let the heat escape and can disrupt the cooking process. If you keep checking your food, you may have to increase the cooking time in the end.

• Don't Be Afraid of Healthy Fat:
These are keto recipes after all, so don't be afraid to use healthy fats! This goes for keto, low carb and paleo diets - healthy fats are necessary. Specifically for the skillet recipes, you will need to cook the recipes in some type of fat, so don't be afraid to do so. Cooking in coconut oil is great because coconut oil is high in saturated fats and will not oxidize and go rancid as quickly in the pan as some of the other oils would.

Cooking
WITH AN INSTANT POT

Another way to make one pot wonders is by using an instant pot. An instant pot has the ability to make recipes that you would traditionally make in a skillet, roasting pan, pressure cooker and slow cooker. Here are some of the functions the instant pot has, to help you get started:

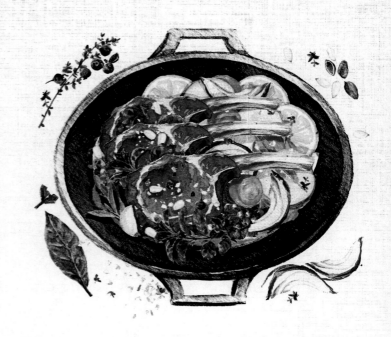

• **Multigrain:**
You will most likely not be using this button much as it's meant for harder grains such as rice, which are not keto friendly!

• **Beans/Chili:**
Although you won't be consuming traditional chili on the ketogenic diet, this setting could work well for a keto-friendly chili made with beef and some non-starchy vegetables.

• **Soup:**
A great setting to make all your low carb soups, fast! You can make both soup and broth using this setting.

• **Sauté:**
You can now make your sautéed dishes in a pot using the instant pot. You can use the instant pot to sauté your meals with the lid open.

• **Slow Cooker:**
If you have an instant pot and not a slow cooker, this setting will be your best friend.

• **Poultry:**
This setting is perfect for your poultry dishes and cooks them quite fast.

• **Steam:**
If you're looking to steam your vegetables, this is a quick and easy setting to do so.

• **Manual:**
If none of the settings make sense for what you are making, the manual setting allows you to set the cooking time.

• **Stew/Meat:**
You can use this setting for things like pot roasts, stews or any type of cooked meat. It only takes about 45 minutes to make a super tender dish.

9

How This Book Works

This cookbook contains helpful cooking tips so that you can make the best one pot recipe possible! There are also serving suggestions listed to give you an idea about what each of these dishes pairs well with. You will also notice there is a difficulty level and cost scale listed on each recipe. Here is how to read both of these scales to determine the difficulty and price scale for each one pot recipe.

Difficulty Level: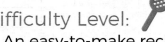

1. An easy-to-make recipe that can be put together with just a handful of ingredients and in a short amount of time.
2. These recipes are a little more difficult and time consuming, but are still easy enough even for beginners.
3. A more advanced recipe for the adventurous cook! You will not see too many level 3 recipes in this book. These recipes are great for when you have a little bit more time to spend in the kitchen and when you want to make something out of the ordinary.

Cost:

$: A-low-budget everyday recipe.

$$: A middle of the road, moderately priced recipe. The majority of the recipes you will find in this book are considered a level $$ on the cost scale.

$$$: A more expensive recipe that is great for serving at a family gathering or party. These recipes tend to contain pricy ingredients such as higher quality meat products. You will not see too many level $$$ recipes in this book, but there are a few that you can make to impress your guests with!

Dietary Labels:

Within this book, you will notice that there are dietary labels. These will indicate whether or not a recipe is gluten free or dairy free. Many recipes can be created dairy free if you remove the added cheese or substitute the milk or cream for coconut milk.

Final Words

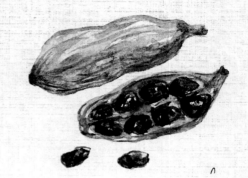

Finally, I want to thank you for purchasing this book and I really hope it helps you keep to your health goals.

If you enjoyed this book or have any suggestions, then I'd appreciate it if you would leave a review or simply email me.

You can leave a review on Amazon at the link below:
http://geni.us/onepotreview

or email me at:
elizabeth@elizjanehealthy.com

Elizabeth

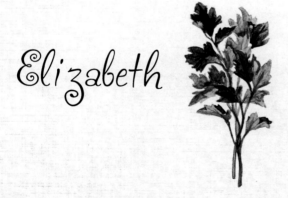

Bonus Keto Sweet Eats

I am delighted you have chosen my book to help you start or continue on your keto journey. Temptation by sweet treats can knock you off course so, to help you stay on the keto track, I am pleased to offer you three mini ebooks from my 'Keto Sweet Eats Series', completely free of charge! These three mini ebooks cover how to make everything from keto chocolate cake to keto ice cream to keto fat bombs so you don't have to feel like you are missing out, whatever the occasion.

Simply visit the link below to get your free copy of all three mini ebooks:

http://genius/onepot

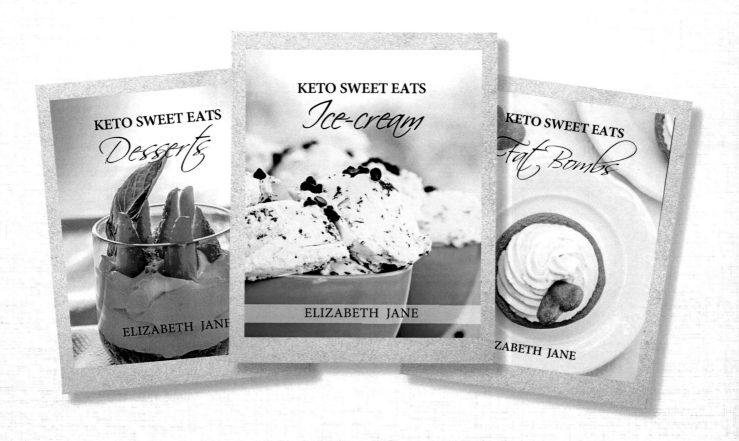

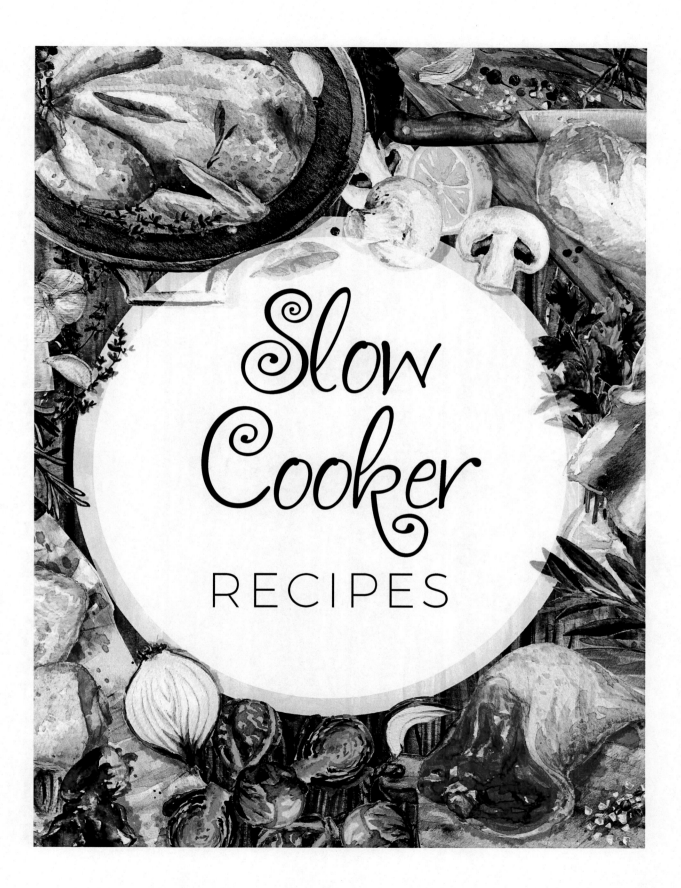

Slow Cooker

RECIPES

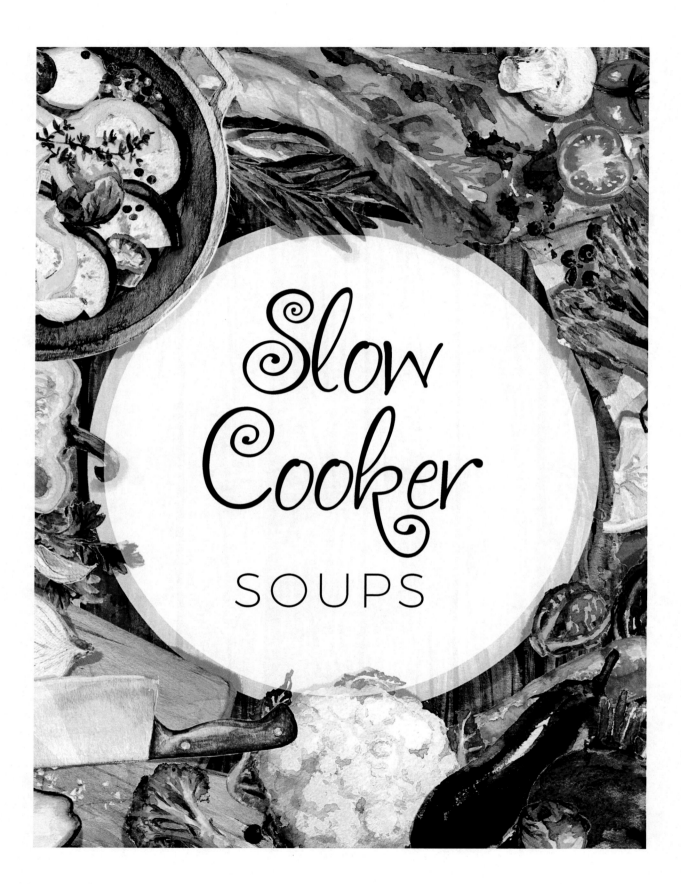

Slow Cooker
SOUPS

Creamy Pumpkin Soup

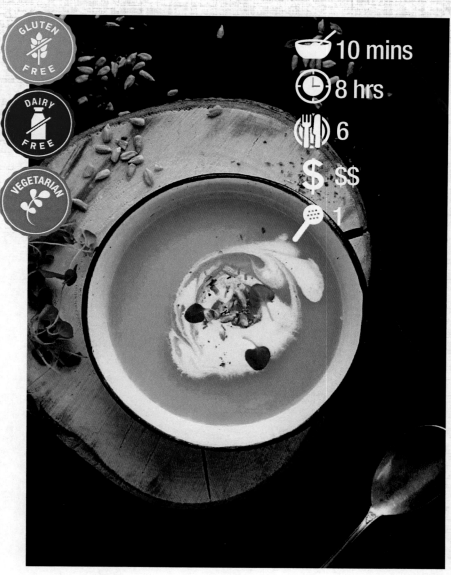

GLUTEN FREE

DAIRY FREE

VEGETARIAN

🥄 10 mins

🕐 8 hrs

🍴 6

$ $$

1

Ingredients:

- 1 (15 oz.) can pure pumpkin puree (unsweetened)
- 1 yellow onion, chopped
- 3 cloves garlic, chopped
- 4 cups reduced sodium vegetable broth
- 1 cup unsweetened full-fat coconut milk
- ½ tsp. ground cinnamon
- ½ tsp. ground nutmeg
- ¼ tsp. cloves
- ¼ tsp. black pepper
- Salt to taste
- Sesame seeds for garnish

Cooking Tips:
Feel free to use heavy cream in place of coconut milk, but note that this recipe would then no longer be considered dairy free.

Serving Suggestions:
Serve with an extra dash of cinnamon if desired.

Directions:

1. Start by adding the vegetable broth, coconut milk and seasonings to the base of a slow cooker and gently stir to combine.

2. Add the remaining ingredients, minus the sesame seeds, and gently stir again.

3. Cook on low for 8 hours.

4. Garnish with sesame seeds to serve.

Nutrition Facts (Per Serving)

Total Carbs 11g   Dietary Fiber 10g   Protein 3g   Total Fat 10g

Net Carbs 1g   Calories 136

% calories from

Fat 63%   Carbs 28%   Protein 8%

15

Russian-
Style Fish
Soup

GLUTEN FREE
DAIRY FREE

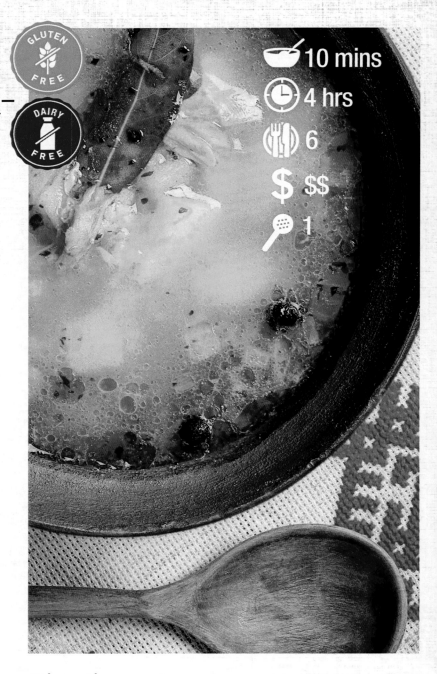

🥣 10 mins
🕐 4 hrs
🍴 6
💲 $$
🥄 1

Ingredients:

- 2 salmon fillets, skin removed and cut into chunks
- 1 onion, chopped
- 2 cloves garlic, chopped
- 2 cups water
- 2 cups reduced sodium vegetable broth
- ½ tsp. black pepper
- 1 tsp. salt
- 2 whole sage leaves

Serving Suggestions:
Serve with a sprinkle of Parmesan cheese if desired. Please note that this soup would no longer be dairy free with the addition of cheese.

Directions:

1. Simply add all of the ingredients to the base of a slow cooker and cook on low for 4 hours.

2. Remove the sage leaves before serving.

Nutrition Facts (Per Serving)

Total Carbs 2g	Dietary Fiber 0g	Protein 29g
Total Fat 8g	Net Carbs 2g	Calories 202

% calories from

Fat 37%   Carbs 4%   Protein 59%

Chicken
Fajita Soup

Ingredients:

- 3 boneless skinless chicken breasts
- 4 cups reduced sodium chicken stock
- 1 (14.5 oz.) can crushed tomatoes
- 1 green pepper, chopped
- 1 yellow onion, chopped
- 3 cloves garlic, chopped
- 1 cup mushrooms, chopped
- 1 tsp. red pepper flakes
- Salt & pepper to taste
- Cilantro for serving

Directions:

1. Add all of the ingredients to the base of the slow cooker.
2. Cook on low for 6 hours.
3. Once cooked, use two forks to shred the chicken.
4. Serve with fresh cilantro.

Nutrition Facts
(Per Serving)

Total Carbs	9g
Dietary Fiber	3g
Protein	22g
Total Fat	3g
Net Carbs	6g
Calories	150

% calories from	
Fat	18%
Carbs	24%
Protein	59%

Cooking Tips:
Check the soup after 2 hours and add a splash more broth if needed.

Serving Suggestions:
Serve with a pinch of red pepper flakes if you want to add more heat.

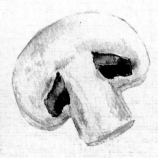

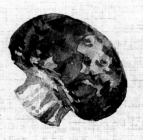

Cream of Mushroom Soup

GLUTEN FREE

VEGETARIAN

🥣 10 mins
🕐 4 hrs
🍴 8
$ $$
🔍 1

Ingredients:

- ½ cup butter
- 1 yellow onion, chopped
- 3 cloves garlic, chopped
- 2 cups mushrooms, sliced
- 4 cups reduced sodium vegetable broth
- 2 cups heavy cream
- 1 tsp. dried marjoram
- 1 tsp. dried basil
- Salt & pepper to taste

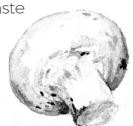

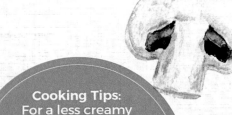

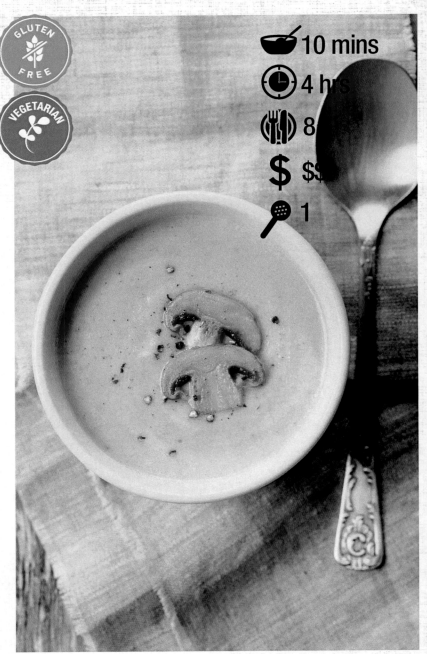

Cooking Tips:
For a less creamy soup, reduce heavy cream to 1 cup and add 1 cup of water.

Serving Suggestions:
Serve with a side salad for lunch and top with herbs of choice if desired.

Directions:

1. Start by adding the butter, garlic and onions to the base of a slow cooker.

2. Add the remaining ingredients and cook on low for 4 hours, stirring at the halfway point.

Nutrition Facts (Per Serving)

| Total Carbs | 4g | Dietary Fiber | 0g | Protein | 3g | Total Fat | 34g |
| Net Carbs | 4g | Calories | 324 | | | | |

% calories from
Fat 93%   Carbs 4%   Protein 3%

Goulash Soup

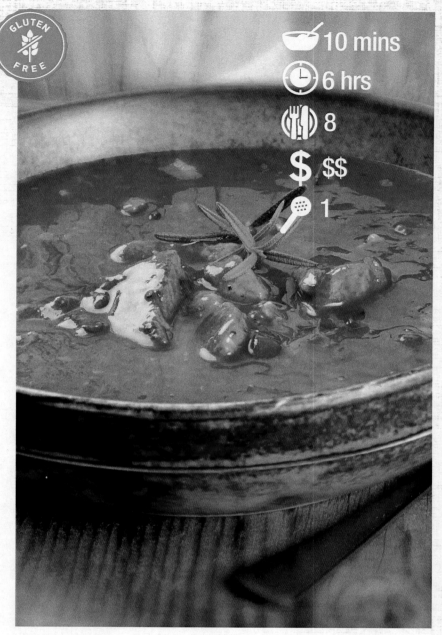

GLUTEN FREE

🥣 10 mins

🕐 6 hrs

🍴 8

$ $$

1

Ingredients:

- 1 lb. boneless steak, cut into cubes
- 1 onion, chopped
- 1 red bell pepper, chopped
- 2 cloves garlic, chopped
- 1 (14.5 oz.) can diced tomatoes
- 3 cups reduced sodium beef broth
- ½ cup water
- ½ cup heavy cream
- Pinch sea salt to taste
- Pinch black pepper to taste

Cooking Tips:
Check the steak at the 5 hour mark; you will know the steak is cooked when it is tender.

Serving Suggestions:
Serve with a dollop of sour cream per serving, if desired.

Directions:

1. Add the steak to the base of the slow cooker with the onion, pepper and garlic.

2. Top the steak with the tomatoes, beef broth, water and heavy cream. Season with salt and pepper.

3. Cook on low for 6 hours.

Nutrition Facts (Per Serving)

Total Carbs 5g   Dietary Fiber 1g   Protein 14g   Total Fat 12g
Net Carbs 4g   Calories 185

% calories from
Fat 58%   Carbs 11%   Protein 30%

Jamaican Style Conch Soup

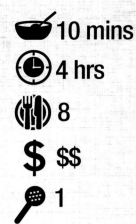

🥣 10 mins
🕐 4 hrs
🍴 8
$ $$
🍳 1

DAIRY FREE · GLUTEN FREE

Ingredients:
- 6 cups reduced sodium chicken broth
- 3 cloves garlic, chopped
- 2 carrots, sliced
- 1 onion, chopped
- 1 green onion, chopped
- 1 hot chili pepper, sliced
- 1 red pepper, sliced
- 1 plum tomato, sliced
- 1 lb. conch meat, cut into small pieces
- 1 cup unsweetened full-fat coconut milk
- 1 tsp. ground cumin
- ¼ tsp. ground ginger
- 1 tsp. salt
- 1 handful fresh cilantro for serving

Directions:
1. Add all of the ingredients to the slow cooker, minus the cilantro, Gently stir to combine.
2. Cook on low for 4 hours, stirring halfway through.
3. Serve with fresh cilantro.

Nutrition Facts
(Per Serving)

Total Carbs	8g
Dietary Fiber	2g
Protein	10g
Total Fat	8g
Net Carbs	6g
Calories	140

% calories from

Fat	50%
Carbs	22%
Protein	28%

Cooking Tips:
Be sure to stir the soup at the halfway point.

Serving Suggestions:
Drizzle with extra coconut milk to serve if desired.

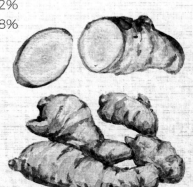

Pepper & Onion Beef Soup

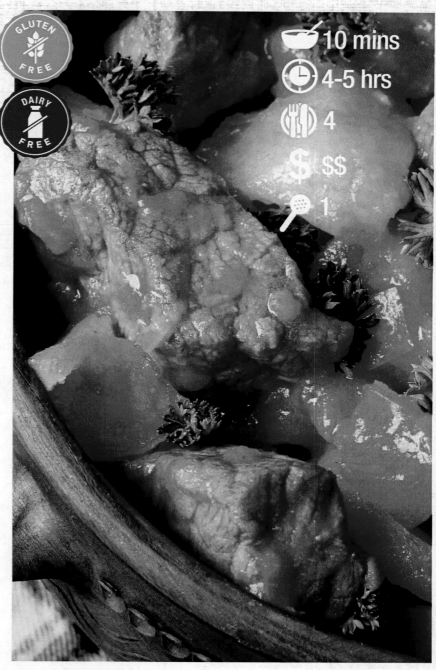

GLUTEN FREE

DAIRY FREE

🥣 10 mins
🕐 4-5 hrs
🍴 4
$ $$
1

Ingredients:

- 1 lb. lean beef chunks
- 4 cups reduced sodium beef broth
- 1 (14.5 oz.) can crushed tomatoes
- 1 red bell pepper, sliced
- 1 yellow onion, chopped
- 3 cloves garlic, chopped
- ½ cup carrots, sliced
- 1 zucchini, cut into rounds
- Salt & pepper to taste

Cooking Tips:
Check the soup after 2 hours and add a splash more beef broth if needed.

Serving Suggestions:
Serve with a sprinkle of Parmesan cheese if desired. Please note that the recipe would no longer be dairy free if you chose to add cheese. You can also add fresh cilantro for serving as well.

Directions:

1. Add all of the ingredients to the base of the slow cooker.
2. Cook on low for 4–5 hours.

Nutrition Facts (Per Serving)

Total Carbs 9g	Dietary Fiber 2g	Protein 17g	Total Fat 13g
Net Carbs 7g	Calories 222		

% calories from

Fat 53%	Carbs 16%	Protein 30%

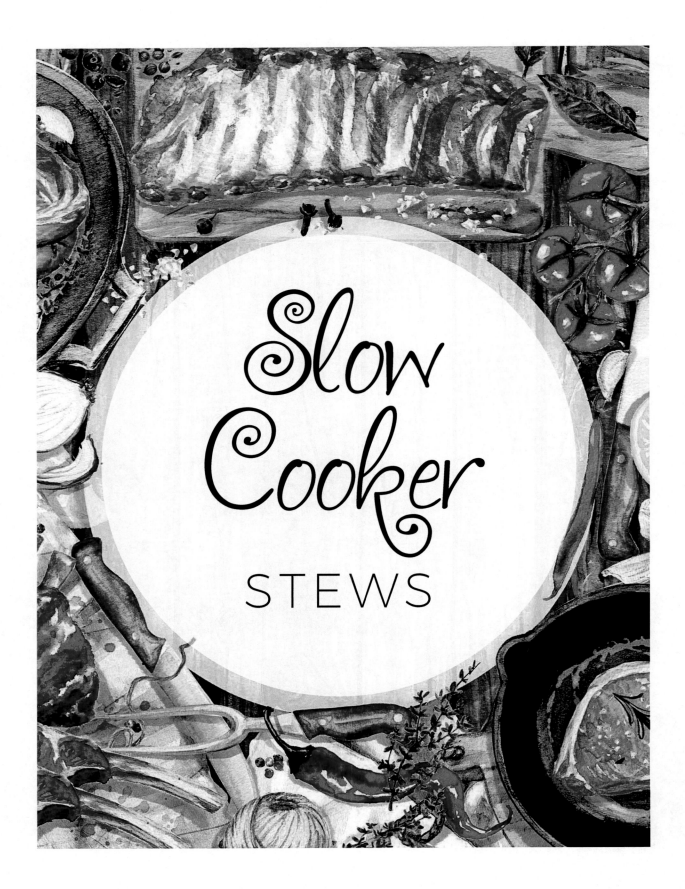

Slow Cooker
STEWS

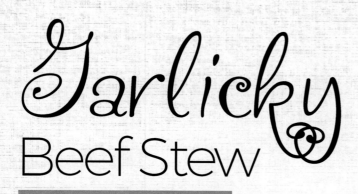

Garlicky Beef Stew

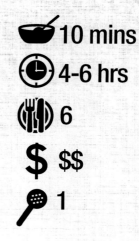

Ingredients:

- 2 lb. beef stew meat, cut into cubes
- ½ cup carrots, sliced
- ½ cup frozen peas
- 1 small white onion, chopped
- 2 green onions, thinly sliced
- 4 cloves garlic, chopped
- ½ tsp. sea salt
- ½ tsp. black pepper
- 1 ½ cups reduced sodium beef broth
- 1 tsp. Worcestershire sauce

Directions:

1. Start by adding the cubed beef to the base of the slow cooker and then top with the veggies.

2. Pour in the beef broth and cook on high for 4–6 hours.

Nutrition Facts
(Per Serving)

Total Carbs	5g
Dietary Fiber	1g
Protein	28g
Total Fat	25g
Net Carbs	4g
Calories	362

% calories from

Fat	62%
Carbs	6%
Protein	31%

Serving Suggestions:
Serve with a side of steamed vegetables such as Brussels sprouts or cauliflower.

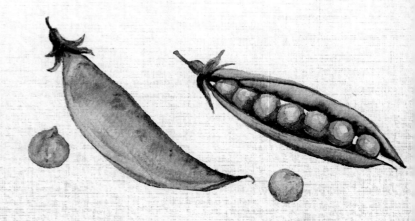

Creamy Mushroom Beef Stew

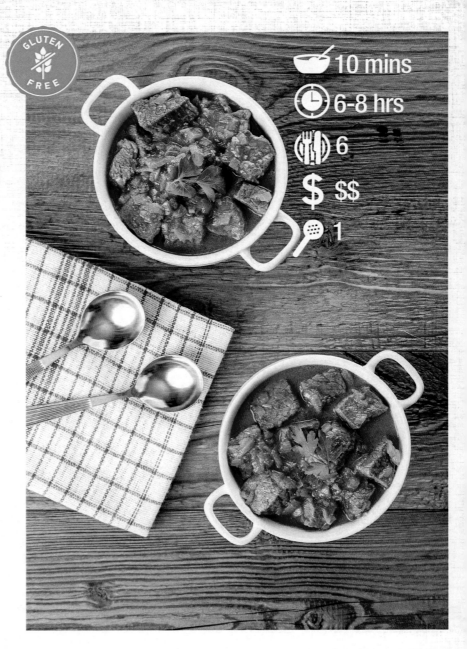

GLUTEN FREE

🥄 10 mins
🕐 6-8 hrs
🍴 6
$ $$
1

Ingredients:

- 2 pounds cubed stew meat
- 1 cup mushrooms, sliced
- 1 onion, sliced
- 4 cloves garlic, chopped
- 1 tsp. onion powder
- 1 tsp. salt
- 1 ½ cup water
- ½ cup heavy cream

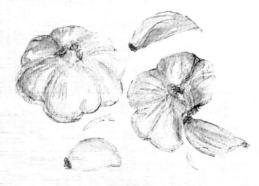

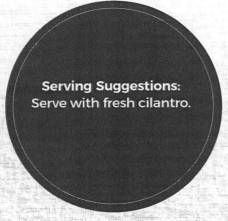

Serving Suggestions:
Serve with fresh cilantro.

Directions:

1. Place all of the ingredients into the base of the slow cooker minus the heavy cream.

2. Cook on low for 6–8 hours or until the beef is cooked through. At the halfway point, add the heavy cream and stir.

Nutrition Facts (Per Serving)

Total Carbs 3g   Dietary Fiber 0g   Protein 32g   Total Fat 24g
Net Carbs 3g   Calories 355

% calories from
Fat 60%   Carbs 4%   Protein 36%

Cinnamon Butternut Beef Stew

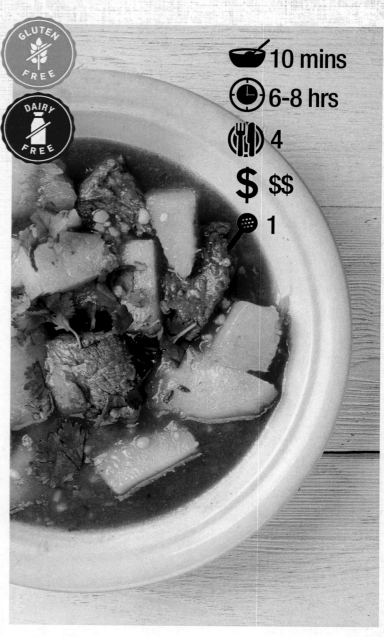

GLUTEN FREE

DAIRY FREE

🥣 10 mins

🕐 6-8 hrs

🍴 4

$ $$

1

Ingredients:

- 1 cup reduced sodium chicken broth
- 1 lb. flank steak, cut into cubes
- 1 cup butternut squash, cubed
- 1 onion, sliced
- 4 cloves garlic, chopped
- 1 tsp. ground cinnamon
- 1 tsp. salt
- 1 tsp. freshly ground black pepper
- Cilantro for serving

Directions:

1. Place all of the ingredients, minus the cilantro, into the base of the slow cooker.

2. Cook on low for 6–8 hours or until the steak is tender and cooked all the way through.

Nutrition Facts (Per Serving)

Total Carbs 8g	Dietary Fiber 2g	Protein 24g
Total Fat 12g	Net Carbs 6g	Calories 240

% calories from

Fat 45%	Carbs 13%	Protein 40%

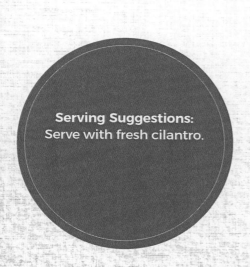

Serving Suggestions:
Serve with fresh cilantro.

Hamburger Stew

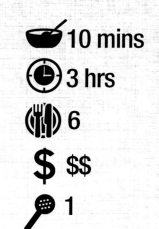

GLUTEN FREE

🍜 10 mins

🕐 3 hrs

🍴 6

$ $$

🥄 1

Ingredients:

- 1 lb. ground beef
- 3 cups reduced sodium beef broth
- 1 cup reduced sodium tomato paste
- 1 tomato, chopped
- 1 yellow onion, chopped
- 3 cloves garlic, chopped
- 1 tsp. garlic powder
- ½ cup shredded American cheese
- Salt & pepper to taste

Directions:

1. Add all of the ingredients to the base of the slow cooker minus the cheese.

2. Cook on high for 3 hours.

3. Once cooked, add the shredded cheese and cook for another 10–15 minutes or until the cheese has melted.

Nutrition Facts
(Per Serving)

Total Carbs	12g
Dietary Fiber	2g
Protein	18g
Total Fat	12g
Net Carbs	10g
Calories	218

% calories from

Fat	47%
Carbs	21%
Protein	32%

Cooking Tips:
Check the slow cooker at the 2 hour mark and stir. Add a splash more broth if needed.

Serving Suggestions:
Add cooked bacon bits for an extra savory flavor.

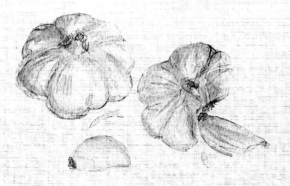

Fire Roasted Vegetable Stew

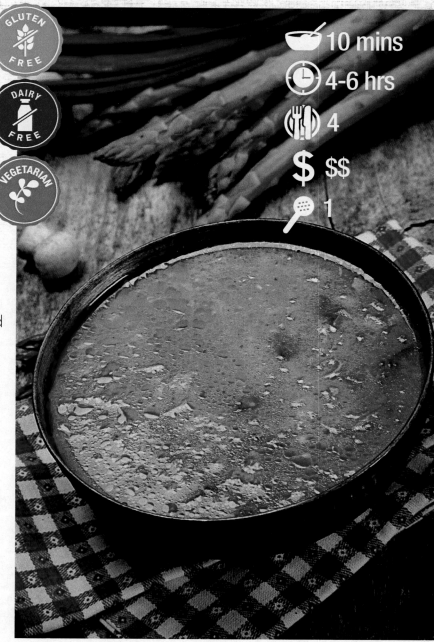

GLUTEN FREE
DAIRY FREE
VEGETARIAN

🥣 10 mins
🕐 4-6 hrs
🍴 4
$ $$
🥄 1

Ingredients:

- 1 medium white onion, chopped
- 2 cloves garlic, chopped
- 3 spears asparagus, finely chopped
- ¼ cup button mushrooms, chopped
- ½ (14.5 oz.) can fire roasted tomatoes
- 2 cups celery, chopped
- 1 cup kale, chopped
- 1 tsp. fresh rosemary
- 1 tsp. fresh oregano
- 1 tsp. paprika
- ½ tsp. salt
- ½ tsp. black pepper
- 5 cups of reduced sodium vegetable broth

Cooking Tips:
Stir halfway through, and add a splash more vegetable broth if needed.

Serving Suggestions:
Serve with a sprinkle of Parmesan cheese if desired but please note that this would no longer be dairy free.

Directions:

1. Simply add all of the vegetables to the base of a slow cooker and cover with the vegetable broth.

2. Cook on high for 4–6 hours.

Nutrition Facts (Per Serving)

Total Carbs 10g	Dietary Fiber 3g	Protein 5g
Total Fat 1g	Net Carbs 7g	Calories 61

% calories from

Fat 13%	Carbs 58%	Protein 29%

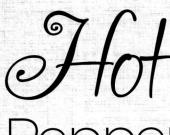

Hot Pepper Chicken Stew

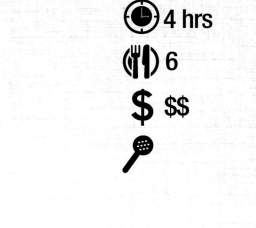

🥣 10 mins

🕐 4 hrs

🍴 6

💲 $$

🥄

Ingredients:

- 6 chicken breasts, cubed
- 1 onion, cubed
- 2 cloves garlic, chopped
- 3 cups reduced sodium chicken broth
- 1 (14.5 oz.) can fire roasted tomatoes
- 1 medium red jalapeño pepper, chopped
- 1 tsp. salt
- 1 tsp. black pepper
- ¼ tsp. chili pepper

Directions:

1. Start by adding the chicken, garlic and onion to the base of the slow cooker and top with the tomatoes, red jalapeño pepper, seasonings and chicken broth.

2. Cook on high for 4 hours.

Nutrition Facts (Per Serving)

Total Carbs	5g
Dietary Fiber	1g
Protein	27g
Total Fat	4g
Net Carbs	4g
Calories	164

% calories from

Fat	22%
Carbs	12%
Protein	66%

Cooking Tips:
Stir halfway through and taste. Adjust seasoning as desired.

Serving Suggestions:
Serve with a side of sautéed kale or a spinach salad.

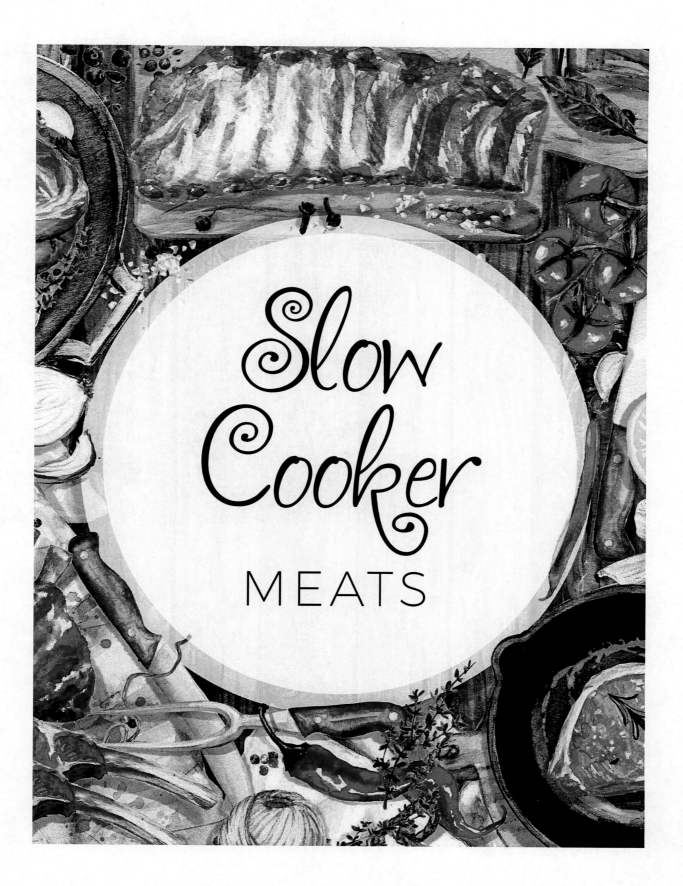

Slow Cooker

MEATS

Rose-mary Peppered Steak

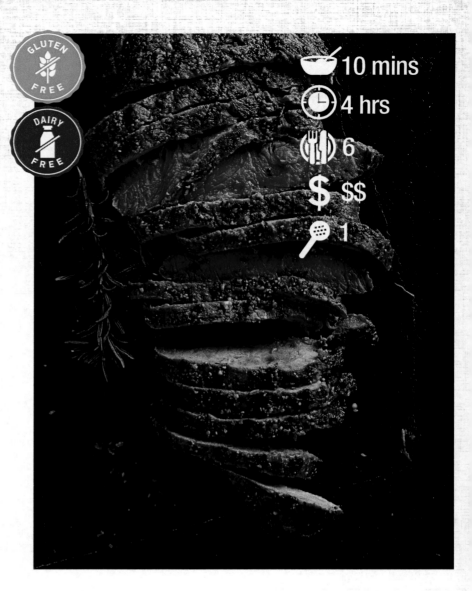

GLUTEN FREE

DAIRY FREE

10 mins
4 hrs
6
$ $$
1

Ingredients:

- 2 lb. beef sirloin steak, cut into strips
- 1 Tbsp. fresh rosemary, chopped
- 2 tsp. garlic powder
- 1 sprig rosemary
- 2 tsp. black pepper
- 1 tsp. salt
- 3 Tbsp. coconut aminos
- ¼ cup water
- 1 cube beef bouillon

Directions:

1. Start by seasoning the steak strips with the garlic, rosemary, salt and pepper.

2. Add the coconut aminos, water and beef bouillon to the slow cooker.

3. Next, add the steak with the rosemary sprig and cook on high for 4 hours.

4. Remove the rosemary sprig before serving.

Serving Suggestions: Serve with a side of sautéed vegetables or serve the steak strips on top of a salad.

Nutrition Facts (Per Serving)

| Total Carbs | 2g | Dietary Fiber | 0g | Protein | 32g |
| Total Fat | 16g | Net Carbs | 2g | Calories | 286 |

% calories from

Fat 51%   Carbs 3%   Protein 46%

BBQ Sirloin Steak

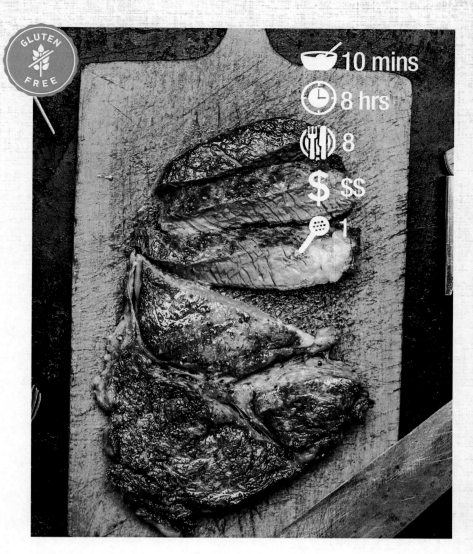

GLUTEN FREE

🥣 10 mins
🕐 8 hrs
🍴 8
$ $$
🔍 1

Ingredients:

- 1 (3 lb.) flank steak
- 1 tsp. granulated garlic
- 1 tsp. granulated onion
- 1 tsp. cayenne pepper
- 1 tsp. paprika
- 1 tsp. white pepper
- 1 tsp. black pepper
- 1 tsp. salt
- 1 Tbsp. coconut aminos
- 2 Tbsp. butter, melted
- ¼ cup water

Directions:

1. Start by adding all of the seasonings, the coconut aminos and the melted butter to a mixing bowl and stir to combine.

2. Rub the seasonings onto the steak.

3. Next, add the water to the base of the slow cooker and then add the steak.

4. Cook on low-medium heat for 8 hours, flipping halfway through. Cook until a fork easily passes through the meat and the steak is tender.

Cooking Tips
At the halfway point, flip the steak and add a splash more water if needed.

Serving Suggestions:
Serve with sautéed spinach, broccoli and caramelized onions.

Nutrition Facts (Per Serving)

Total Carbs 1g	Dietary Fiber 0g	Protein 35g
Total Fat 21g	Net Carbs 1g	Calories 342

% calories from

Fat 57%	Carbs 1%	Protein 42%

Creamy Chicken & Sausage

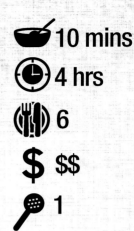

🥣 10 mins

🕐 4 hrs

🍴 6

$ $$

🥄 1

GLUTEN FREE

Ingredients:

- 1 lb. boneless skinless chicken breasts
- 1 (8 oz.) package sausage
- 1 (8 oz.) package cream cheese
- 1 ½ cups reduced sodium chicken broth
- 3 cloves garlic, chopped
- 1 small onion, chopped
- 1 pinch of sea salt & pepper

Directions:

1. Start by putting the cream cheese and chicken broth in a large mixing bowl. Whisk to combine.

2. Place the chicken and sausage into the base of the slow cooker and top with the onion and garlic.

3. Pour the cream cheese mixture on top and add the pinch of salt and pepper.

4. Cook on high for 4 hours or on low for 5–6 hours.

5. Once cooked, cut the chicken and sausage to your liking.

Cooking Tips
Check the slow cooker every hour to make sure that the sauce is not thickening up too much. If it is, add a splash or two more of chicken broth to thin.

Serving Suggestions:
Serve with a side salad or steamed vegetables.

Nutrition Facts
(Per Serving)

Total Carbs	3g
Dietary Fiber	0g
Protein	21g
Total Fat	25g
Net Carbs	3g
Calories	325

% calories from

Fat	69%
Carbs	5%
Protein	26%

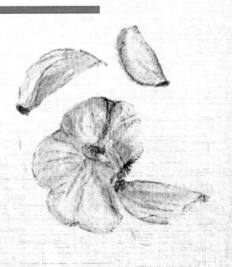

Italian
Beef

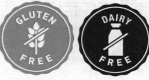

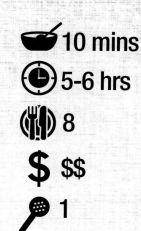

🥣 10 mins

🕐 5-6 hrs

🍴 8

$ $$

🍳 1

Ingredients:

- 2 lb. ground beef
- 1 cup carrots, chopped
- 1 white onion, diced
- 5 cloves garlic, chopped
- 1 Tbsp. Italian seasoning
- ¼ tsp. ground cinnamon
- 1 small pinch red pepper flakes
- 1 (14.5 oz.) can crushed tomatoes
- 2 cups reduced sodium beef broth

Directions:

1. Simply place all of the ingredients into a slow cooker, adding the ground beef to the base first and topping it with the onion, garlic, tomatoes and seasonings.

2. Cook for 5-6 hours on low.

Nutrition Facts
(Per Serving)

Total Carbs	6g
Dietary Fiber	2g
Protein	20g
Total Fat	12g
Net Carbs	4g
Calories	213

% calories from

Fat	51%
Carbs	11%
Protein	38%

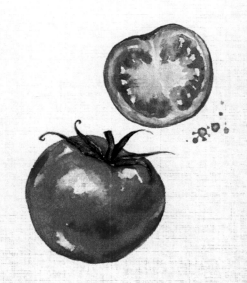

Cooking Tips
Check the slow cooker every hour to make sure that the sauce is not thickening up too much. If it is, add a splash or two more of beef broth to thin.

Serving Suggestions:
Serve with cooked spaghetti squash.

Zesty Meat-balls

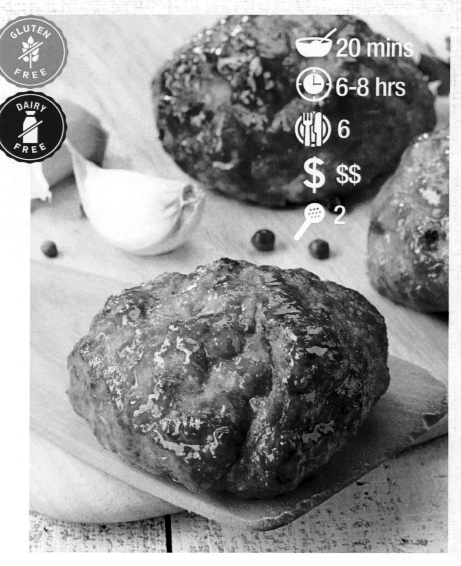

GLUTEN FREE

DAIRY FREE

🥣 20 mins
🕐 6-8 hrs
🍴 6
$ $$
🧂 2

Ingredients:

- 2 lb. ground beef
- 1 egg, lightly beaten
- ½ cup tomato paste
- 1 (14.5 oz.) can diced tomatoes
- 2 cloves garlic, chopped
- 1 Tbsp. Italian seasoning
- 1 tsp. freshly ground black pepper
- 1 tsp. red pepper flakes
- ¼ cup water

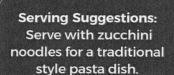

Serving Suggestions:
Serve with zucchini noodles for a traditional style pasta dish.

Directions:

1. Add all of the ingredients minus the water and diced tomatoes to a large mixing bowl and stir to combine.

2. Shape into 12 meatballs.

3. Add the water and diced tomatoes to the base of a slow cooker and place the meatballs on top.

4. Cook on low for 6–8 hours until cooked through.

Nutrition Facts (Per Serving)

Total Carbs 7g   Dietary Fiber 2g   Protein 24g   Total Fat 16g
Net Carbs   5g   Calories 271

% calories from
Fat   54%   Carbs   10%   Protein   36%

Lemon & Herb Whole Chicken

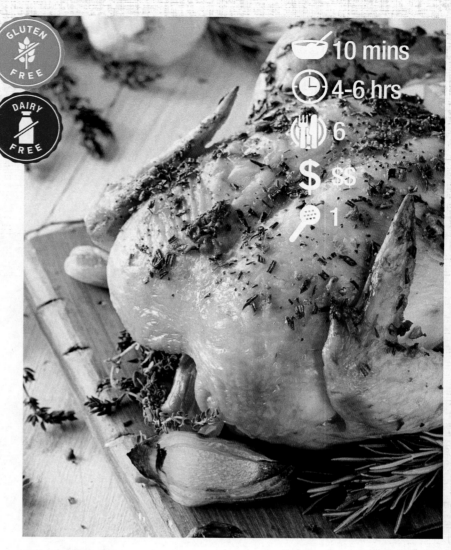

GLUTEN FREE

DAIRY FREE

10 mins
4-6 hrs
6
$ $$
1

Ingredients:

- 1 whole (4 lb.) chicken
- 2 lemon wedges, sliced
- 4 cloves garlic, chopped
- 2 sprigs rosemary
- 1 tsp. dried thyme
- 1 tsp. onion powder
- ¼ tsp. black pepper
- 1 tsp. salt

Directions:

1. Start by mixing the thyme, onion powder, salt and pepper together in a small mixing bowl.

2. Rub the seasonings over the whole chicken and place the chicken into the slow cooker with the garlic, lemon wedges and rosemary sprigs.

3. Cook on low for 4–6 hours or until the juices run clear.

4. Remove the rosemary sprigs and lemon wedges before serving.

Cooking Tips:
Check the chicken at the 4-hour mark. If the juices still aren't clear, continue to cook.

Serving Suggestions:
Squeeze extra lemon juice over the chicken before serving for an extra zesty flavor.

Nutrition Facts (Per Serving)

Total Carbs 1g   Dietary Fiber 0g   Protein 34g   Total Fat 31g
Net Carbs 1g   Calories 428

% calories from
Fat 67%   Carbs 1%   Protein 32%

Italian
Chicken
Parmesan

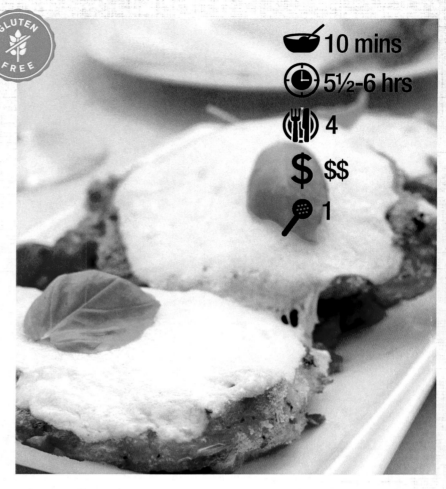

GLUTEN FREE

🍲 10 mins

🕐 5½-6 hrs

🍴 4

$ $$

🔍 1

Ingredients:

- 4 boneless skinless chicken breasts
- 1 (14.5 oz.) can crushed tomatoes
- 1 Tbsp. Italian seasoning
- 1 cup shredded full fat mozzarella cheese
- ½ cup grated Parmesan cheese
- 2 Tbsp. olive oil
- Fresh basil for garnish

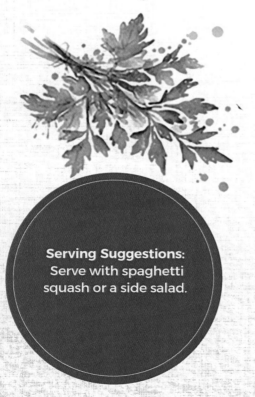

Serving Suggestions:
Serve with spaghetti squash or a side salad.

Directions:

1. Start by mixing the olive oil and seasoning together. Rub the mixture onto the chicken breasts.

2. Add the chicken to the slow cooker, followed by the can of crushed tomatoes, followed by the Parmesan and, finally, the mozzarella, laying the mozzarella carefully on top of the chicken breasts.

3. Cook on low for 5 ½–6 hours.

4. Gently remove the chicken breasts from the slow cooker and top each one with a garnish of fresh basil.

Nutrition Facts (Per Serving)

Total Carbs 5g   Dietary Fiber 2g   Protein 38g   Total Fa 18g

Net Carbs 3g   Calories 336

% calories from

Fat 48%   Carbs 6%   Protein 45%

Peanut Curried Chicken

GLUTEN FREE
DAIRY FREE

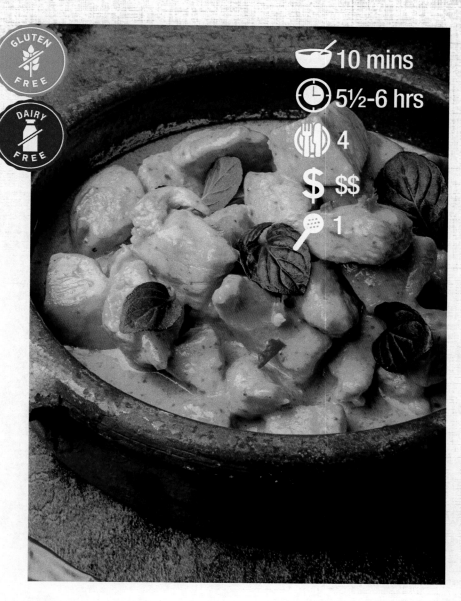

🥣 10 mins
🕐 5½-6 hrs
🍴 4
$ $$
1

Ingredients:

- 4 boneless skinless chicken breasts, cubed
- 1 cup unsweetened full-fat coconut milk
- 1 tsp. curry powder
- 1 tsp. curry paste
- 2 Tbsp. peanut butter
- 2 Tbsp. coconut aminos
- 1 yellow onion, chopped
- 1 red bell pepper, sliced
- Spicy red chili pepper, chopped for garnish

Directions:

1. Start by whisking together the coconut milk, curry paste, curry powder, peanut butter and coconut aminos in the base of the slow cooker.

2. Next, add the remaining ingredients and cook on high for 5 ½–6 hours.

3. Garnish with spicy red pepper.

Cooking Tips:
Check to be sure the coconut milk is not thickening up too much during cooking time. If it is, add a splash or two of water and stir.
Serving Suggestions:
Serve with steamed snap peas or cauliflower and garnish with fresh basil if desired.

Nutrition Facts (Per Serving)

Total Carbs 9g   Dietary Fiber 3g   Protein 31g   Total Fat 22g
Net Carbs 6g   Calories 348

% calories from
Fat   55%   Carbs 10%   Protein   35%

Chicken Teriyaki

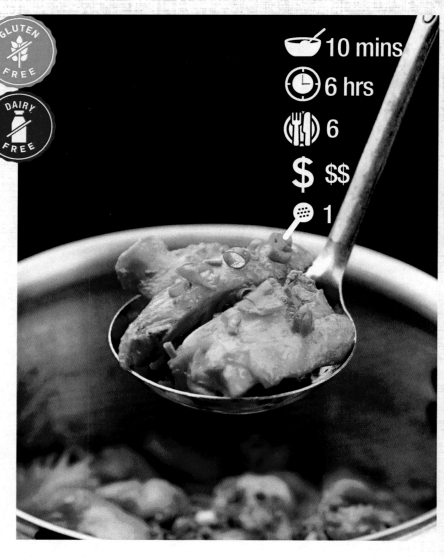

GLUTEN FREE

DAIRY FREE

🥣 10 mins
🕐 6 hrs
🍴 6
$ $$
1

Ingredients:

- 2 lb. chicken thighs
- 1 yellow onion, chopped
- 1 spicy red pepper, chopped
- 3 cloves garlic, chopped
- ¼ cup coconut aminos
- ½ cup reduced sodium beef broth
- ⅓ cup water
- 1 inch knob fresh ginger, grated
- Salt & pepper to taste
- 4 green onions, chopped for garnish
- Lettuce leaves for serving (optional)

Directions:

1. Start by whisking together the coconut aminos, broth and water. Add to the base of the slow cooker with the remaining ingredients, minus the chopped green onions and lettuce.

2. Cook on high for 6 hours.

3. Once cooked, garnish with the chopped green onion and serve with lettuce leaves to form a taco if desired.

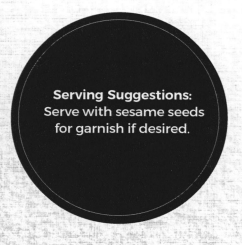

Serving Suggestions:
Serve with sesame seeds for garnish if desired.

Nutrition Facts (Per Serving)

Total Carbs 5g   Dietary Fiber 1g   Protein 20g   Total Fat 6g
Net Carbs 4g   Calories 158

% calories from
Fat   34%   Carbs   13%   Protein   51%

Pepper-corn & Sage Pork Loin

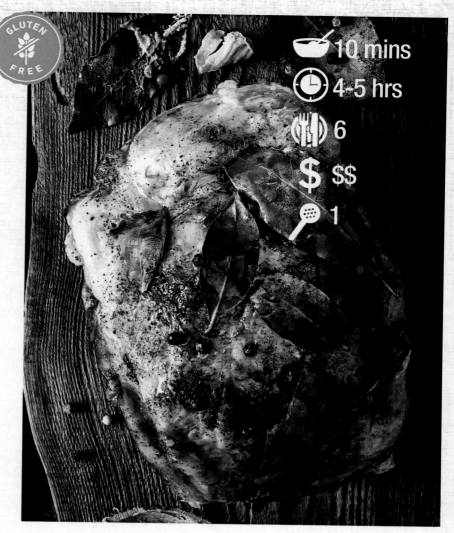

GLUTEN FREE

🥣 10 mins

🕐 4-5 hrs

🍴 6

$ $$

🍳 1

Ingredients:

- 1 (2 lb.) pork tenderloin
- 3 cloves garlic
- 1 Tbsp. onion, minced
- 1 tsp. peppercorn
- ½ tsp. cloves
- ¼ tsp. butter, melted
- 6 sage leaves
- Salt to taste
- 1 ¾ cup water

Directions:

1. Pour the melted butter over the pork and rub with the cloves, peppercorn, garlic, salt and sage leaves.

2. Add the water to the slow cooker and then add the pork.

3. Top with the onion and cook on low for 4-5 hours or until cooked through.

4. Remove the sage leaves before serving and enjoy.

Cooking Tips:
At the halfway point, check the pork and add a splash more water if necessary.

Serving Suggestions:
Serve with a slab of butter if desired.

Nutrition Facts (Per Serving)

Total Carbs 1g   Dietary Fiber 0g   Protein 10g   Total Fat 13g
Net Carbs 1g   Calories 164

% calories from

Fat 73%   Carbs 2%   Protein 25%

Thousand
Island Pork Loin

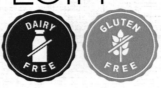

Ingredients:

- 1 (2 lb.) pork tenderloin
- 3 cloves garlic
- 1 Tbsp. onion, minced
- 1 Tbsp. chili sauce
- 2 Tbsp. sweet pickle relish (gluten free)
- 3 Tbsp. coconut aminos
- Salt & pepper to taste
- 1 ¾ cup water

Directions:

1. Start by rubbing the pork with the chili sauce, sweet pickle relish, salt and pepper.

2. Place the pork into the base of a slow cooker and top with the water, garlic, onion and coconut aminos.

3. Cook on low for 4–5 hours or until cooked through.

4. Serve with the cooking liquid and enjoy.

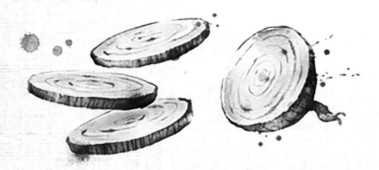

Nutrition Facts
(Per Serving)

Total Carbs	2g
Dietary Fiber	0g
Protein	24g
Total Fat	4g
Net Carbs	2g
Calorie	141

% calories from

Fat	25%
Carbs	6%
Protein	68%

Cooking Tips:
Check the pork at the halfway point and add more liquid if desired.

Serving Suggestions:
Serve with extra chili sauce for a spicier flavor.

Hickory
Baby Back Ribs

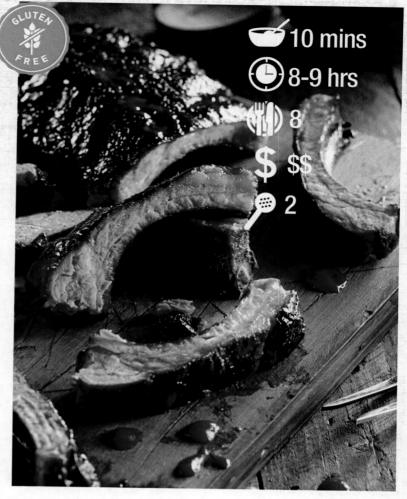

GLUTEN FREE

🥣 10 mins

🕐 8-9 hrs

🍴 8

$ $$

2

Ingredients:

- 3 lb. baby back ribs, trimmed
- 2 cloves garlic, minced
- 1 whole serving of homemade BBQ sauce
- Salt & pepper to taste
- ½ cup water

Homemade BBQ Sauce

- 2 Tbsp. butter
- 1 cup low carb ketchup
- 1 Tbsp. apple cider vinegar
- 2 Tbsp. tomato paste
- ¼ tsp. allspice
- 1 tsp. chili pepper
- 1 tsp. garlic powder
- 1 tsp. onion powder
- ¼ tsp. salt
- ¼ tsp. pepper

Cooking Tips:
Check the ribs at the halfway mark and add more water if necessary.

Serving Suggestions:
Serve with sautéed onions if desired.

Directions:

1. Start by making the homemade BBQ sauce by placing all of the Homemade BBQ sauce ingredients into a mixing bowl.

2. Then, season the ribs with the salt and pepper.

3. Next, put the ribs in a large mixing bowl and add the BBQ sauce. Toss to combine.

4. Add the ribs to the slow cooker, followed by the water and cook on low for 8–9 hours or until they are thoroughly cooked.

Nutrition Facts (Per Serving)

Total Carbs 9g	Dietary Fiber 0g	Protein 30g
Total Fat 20g	Net Carbs 9g	Calories 344

% calories from

Fat 54%	Carbs 11%	Protein 36%

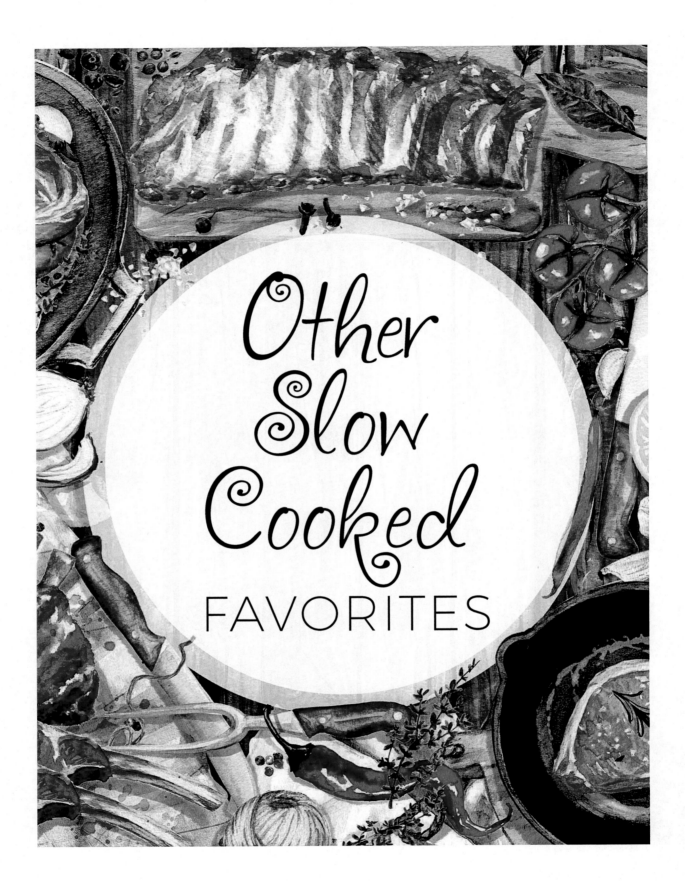

Other
Slow
Cooked
FAVORITES

Southwest Tacos with Coconut Tortillas

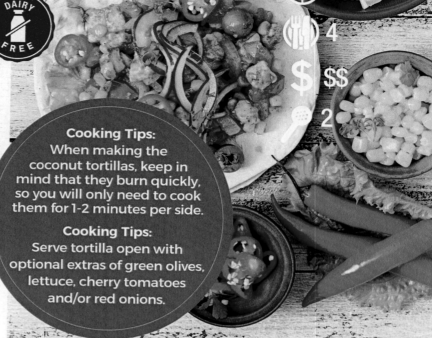

GLUTEN FREE

DAIRY FREE

20 mins

4 hrs

4

$ $$

2

Ingredients:

- 4 chicken breasts, cut into cubes
- 1 tsp. chili powder
- 1 tsp. garlic powder
- 1 tsp. onion powder
- 1 small red chili pepper, sliced
- ¼ cup canned corn
- 1 red onion, sliced
- ¼ cup water
- 4 coconut tortillas for serving

Coconut Tortilla

Serves: 4

Ingredients:

- ¼ cup coconut flour, sifted
- 2 eggs
- ½ cup unsweetened full-fat coconut milk
- 1 Tbsp. coconut oil for cooking

Cooking Tips:
When making the coconut tortillas, keep in mind that they burn quickly, so you will only need to cook them for 1-2 minutes per side.

Cooking Tips:
Serve tortilla open with optional extras of green olives, lettuce, cherry tomatoes and/or red onions.

Directions:

1. Start by adding all of the taco filling ingredients to the base of the slow cooker with the water.

2. Cook on high for 4 hours or until the chicken is cooked through.

3. While the tacos filling is cooking, make the coconut tortillas.

4. Whisk all of the coconut tortilla ingredients together in a large mixing bowl. Let the batter sit for 5 minutes before cooking.

5. While the batter is sitting out, heat the coconut oil in a large skillet over low to medium heat. Pour ¼ of the mixture into the pan and cook for 1-2 minutes on each side until the sides begin to brown. Repeat 3 more times with the remaining mixture.

6. Once the taco filling is cooked through, serve with coconut tortillas (1 tortilla per serving).

Nutrition Facts (Per Serving)

Total Carbs 13g   Dietary Fiber 5g   Protein 31g   Total Fat 17g   Net Carbs 8g   Calories 330

% calories from: Fat 46%   Carbs 16%   Protein 38%

Stuffed Collard Greens

GLUTEN FREE

DAIRY FREE

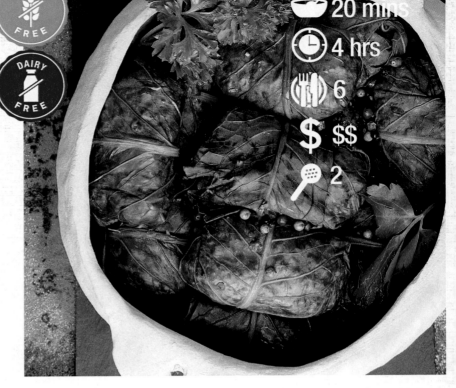

20 mins

4 hrs

6

$ $$

2

Ingredients:

- 1 lb. sirloin steak, thinly sliced
- 1 yellow onion, chopped
- 2 cloves garlic, chopped
- 12 large collard green leaves
- 1 cup reduced sodium beef stock
- ½ cup tomato sauce
- 1 tsp. coconut aminos
- Salt & pepper to taste

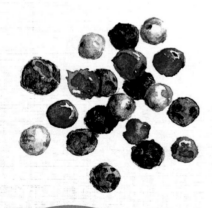

Serving Suggestions: Garnish with peppercorn and fresh parsley. Serve with 1 tsp. of tomato paste spread on top of each wrap, if desired.

Directions:

1. Start by rinsing the collard green leaves and patting them dry.

2. Evenly distribute the sirloin steak, onion and garlic in the center of each leaf, fold the bottom pieces up then fold in the sides and roll to form a collard green wrap.

3. Add half of the stock and half of the tomato sauce to the bottom of the slow cooker and then add the collard green leaves.

4. Pour in the remaining stock and tomato sauce as well as the coconut aminos.

5. Cook on low for 4 hours.

6. Season with salt and pepper to taste.

Nutrition Facts (Per Serving)

Total Carbs 4g   Dietary Fiber 1g   Protein 17g   Total Fat 9g
Net Carbs 3g   Calories 163

% calories from
Fat 50%   Carbs 10%   Protein 40%

Wild Dill Salmon

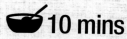 10 mins

 2 hrs

 4

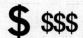 $$$

 1

 GLUTEN FREE

 DAIRY FREE

Ingredients:

- 2 lbs. skin-on wild caught salmon
- 2 cups water
- 1 cup reduced sodium vegetable broth
- 1 lemon, thinly sliced
- 1 onion, finely chopped
- 3 sprigs dill
- Salt & pepper to taste

Directions:

1. Simply place all of the ingredients into a slow cooker, adding the salmon to the base of the slow cooker and then adding the remaining ingredients.

2. Cook for 2 hours on high or until the fish begins to flake.

Nutrition Facts
(Per Serving)

Total Carbs	3g
Dietary Fiber	1g
Protein	50g
Total Fat	13g
Net Carbs	2g
Calories	341

% calories from

Fat	36%
Carbs	4%
Protein	61%

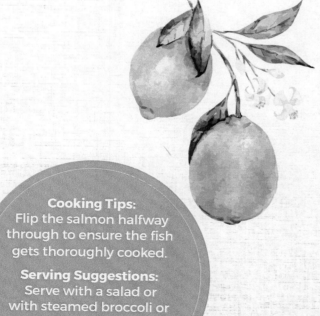

Cooking Tips:
Flip the salmon halfway through to ensure the fish gets thoroughly cooked.

Serving Suggestions:
Serve with a salad or with steamed broccoli or green beans. Add an extra squeeze of fresh lemon juice if desired.

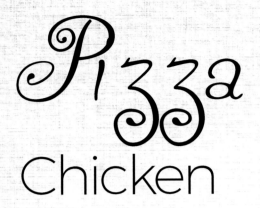

Pizza Chicken

10 mins

6 hrs

4

$ $$

1

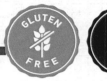

Ingredients:

- 2 boneless skinless chicken breasts
- 1 cup no sugar added marinara sauce
- ½ cup pepperoni, chopped
- 1 yellow onion, chopped
- 3 cloves garlic, chopped
- 1 cup mushrooms, chopped
- 1 tsp. red pepper flakes
- 1 Tbsp. Italian seasoning
- Salt & pepper to taste
- 1 cup of shredded cheese of choice

Directions:

1. Add all of the ingredients to the base of the slow cooker minus the cheese.

2. Cook on low for 6 hours.

3. Once cooked, use a fork to shred the chicken and sprinkle with the shredded cheese.

Nutrition Facts
(Per Serving)

Total Carbs	10g
Dietary Fiber	2g
Protein	23g
Total Fat	16g
Net Carbs	8g
Calories	275

% calories from

Fat	52%
Carbs	15%
Protein	33%

Serving Suggestions:
Serve with shredded mozzarella cheese for an authentic pizza flavor.

Chicken Stuffed Peppers

GLUTEN FREE
DAIRY FREE

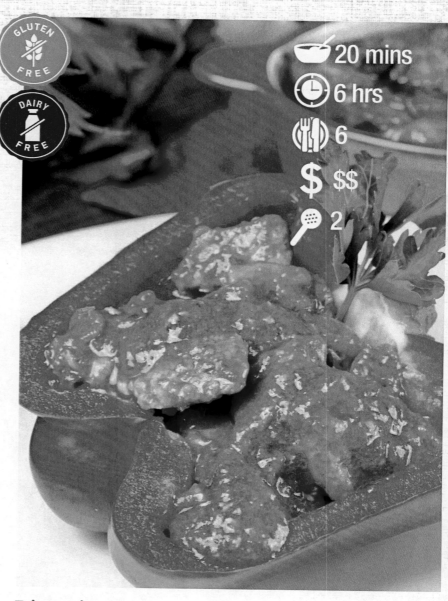

🥄 20 mins
🕐 6 hrs
🍴 6
$ $$
🔍 2

Ingredients:

- 6 chicken breasts, cubed
- 1 cup cauliflower, finely blended
- 1 (14.5 oz.) can fire roasted tomatoes
- 1 tsp. Worcestershire sauce
- 2 Tbsp. tomato paste
- 1 tsp. salt
- 1 tsp. black pepper
- 1 tsp. red pepper flakes
- 6 red bell peppers, tops and seeds removed and sliced in half
- ⅓ cup water

Directions:

1. Start by adding all of the ingredients minus the bell peppers to the slow cooker.

2. Cook on low for 6 hours, stirring halfway through.

3. Once the chicken is thoroughly cooked, scoop the chicken mixture into the pepper halves and enjoy right away!

Cooking Tips:
Check the chicken mixture at the halfway point. If the sauce is becoming too thick, add a splash of water and stir.

Serving Suggestions:
Serve with a sprinkle of shredded cheese if desired. Please note that adding cheese would mean that this recipe would no longer be dairy free.

Nutrition Facts (Per Serving)

Total Carbs 14g	Dietary Fiber 5g	Protein 29g
Total Fat 4g	Net Carbs 9g	Calories 209

% calories from

Fat 17%   Carbs 27%   Protein 56%

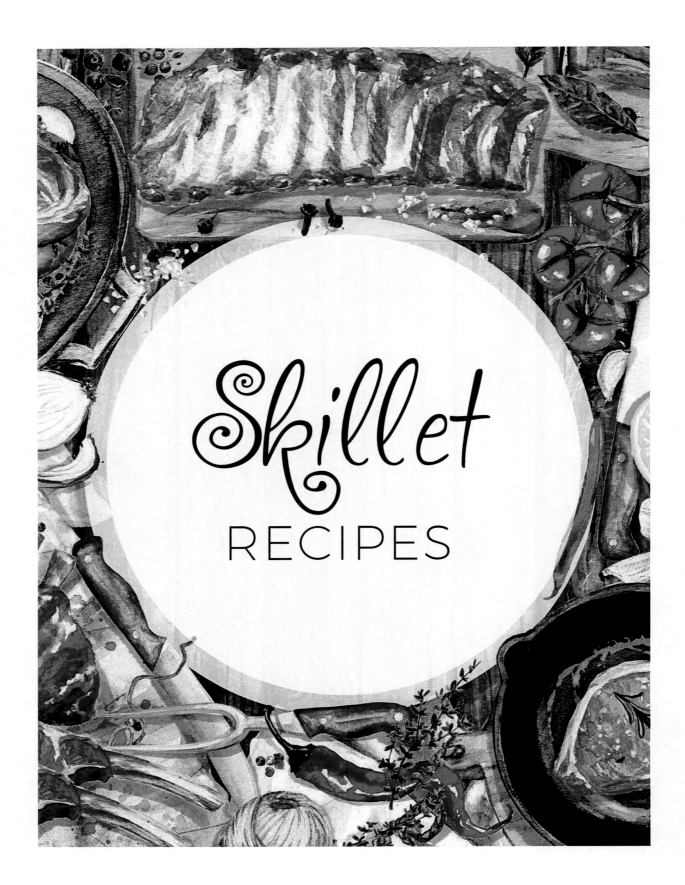

Minced
Meat with Coconut Flour Tortillas

GLUTEN FREE

DAIRY FREE

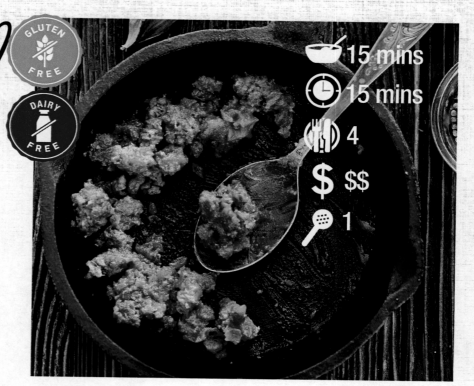

🥣 15 mins

🕐 15 mins

🍴 4

$ $$

🔍 1

Coconut Flour Tortilla Ingredients:

- ¼ cup coconut flour, sifted
- 2 eggs
- ½ cup unsweetened full-fat coconut milk
- 1 Tbsp. coconut oil for cooking

Minced Meat Filling Ingredients:

- 1 lb. ground beef
- 4 Tbsp. tomato paste
- 1 tsp. cumin
- 1 tsp. paprika
- ½ tsp. black peppercorn, ground
- ½ tsp. salt
- 1 Tbsp. coconut oil

Directions:

1. Whisk all of the coconut tortilla ingredients together in a large mixing bowl. Let the batter sit for 5 minutes before cooking.

2. While the batter is sitting out, heat the coconut oil in a large skillet over low to medium heat. Pour a quarter of the mixture into the pan and cook for 1–2 minutes on each side until the sides begin to brown. Repeat this step with the remaining mixture.

3. Wipe a large skillet clean with paper towels and place over medium heat with the coconut oil from the minced meat filling ingredients.

4. Add the ground beef, tomato paste and seasonings into the skillet, and stir to combine.

5. Cook for 7–10 minutes or until the ground beef is cooked through.

6. Split into 4 servings, and serve with a coconut tortilla.

Nutrition Facts (Per Serving)

Total Carbs 10g   Dietary Fiber 4g   Protein 22g   Total Fat 29g   Net Carbs 6g   Calories 378

% calories from   Fat 69%   Carbs 11%   Protein 23%

Filet
With Chive Butter

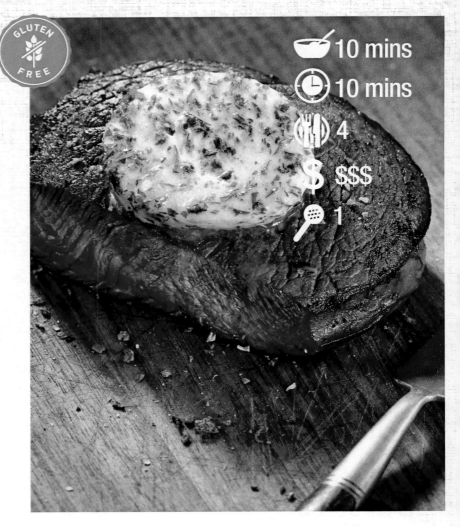

GLUTEN FREE

🥣 10 mins
🕐 10 mins
🍴 4
$ $$$
1

Ingredients:

- 4 (8 oz.) filet mignon steaks
- 1 whole stick (½ cup) butter
- 1 bunch chives, chopped
- 1 clove garlic, chopped
- 2 Tbsp. coconut oil
- 1 tsp. salt
- 1 tsp. pepper

Directions:

1. Start by making the chive butter by adding the butter, chives and garlic to a food processor. Pulse to combine.

2. Next, heat the coconut oil over medium heat, add the filet steaks and cook to your liking. Medium-rare should take about 5–7 minutes each side. Season with salt and pepper.

3. Serve each filet with a slab of the chive butter.

Cooking Tips:
Adjust the cooking time according to how you like your steak cooked.
Serving Suggestions:
Serve with sautéed asparagus or Brussels sprouts.

Nutrition Facts (Per Serving)

Total Carbs 2g   Dietary Fiber 1g   Protein 49g   Total Fat 49g
Net Carbs 1g   Calories 650

% calories from
Fat 68%   Carbs 1%   Protein 30%

Chicken & Steak Mexican Fajita Filling

GLUTEN FREE

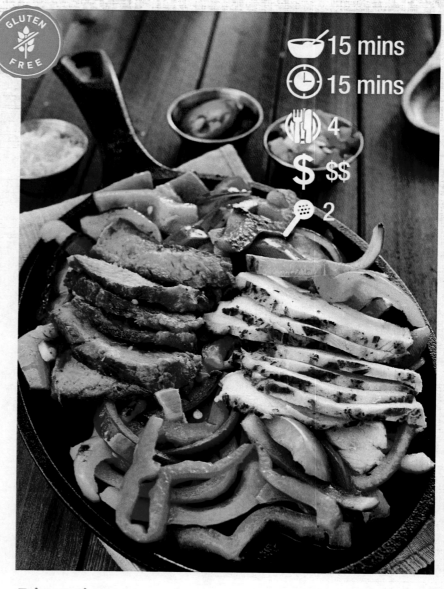

15 mins
15 mins
4
$ $$
2

Ingredients:

- ½ pound steak, thinly sliced
- 2 chicken breasts, thinly sliced
- 1 green pepper, sliced
- 1 red pepper, sliced
- 1 yellow pepper, sliced
- 1 red onion, sliced
- 1 green chili pepper, sliced
- 1 tsp. salt
- 1 tsp. pepper
- 1 tsp. paprika
- ½ cup shredded cheddar cheese
- 2 Tbsp. coconut oil

Serving Suggestions: Increase the paprika for a spicier dish and serve with a homemade coconut tortilla if desired.

Directions:

1. Begin by heating a large skillet over medium heat with the coconut oil. Add the chopped steak and chicken, and sauté for about 7–9 minutes or until cooked through.

2. Add the vegetables and seasonings, and sauté for another 3–5 minutes.

3. Serve with shredded cheddar cheese.

Nutrition Facts (Per Serving)

Total Carbs 7g   Dietary Fiber 2g   Protein 29g   Total Fat 19g
Net Carbs 5g   Calories 318

% calories from
Fat 54%   Carbs 9%   Protein 36%

Herbed
Pan Roasted Chicken Legs

GLUTEN FREE

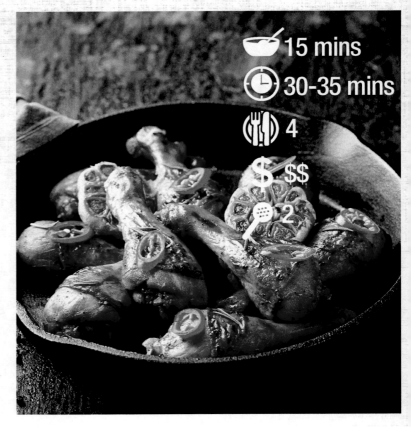

🥣 15 mins

🕐 30-35 mins

🍴 4

$ $$

▦ 2

Ingredients:

- 10 skin-on drumsticks
- 4 Tbsp. butter
- 1 whole head garlic, skin removed and top removed
- 2 tsp. fresh rosemary
- 1 small red chili pepper, sliced
- 1 tsp. salt
- 1 tsp. pepper
- 2 Tbsp. coconut oil

Cooking Tips:
If you find that the drumsticks are not browning when you first add them to the pan, add a tablespoon or two more butter.

Serving Suggestions:
Serve with a side of sautéed vegetables or with a salad.

Directions:

1. Start by seasoning the drumsticks with salt and pepper and heating a large skillet over medium heat.

2. Add the butter to the pan and then add the drumsticks, turning them until they are lightly brown all over. Reduce the heat to low and add the coconut oil.

3. Add the garlic, rosemary and chili pepper. Cover the pan with the lid and cook for another 20–25 minutes, being sure to flip the drumsticks every 5–10 minutes.

4. After the chicken is thoroughly cooked through, remove the lid and let the chicken sit in the pan for another 10 minutes.

Nutrition Facts (Per Serving)

Total Carbs 3g	Dietary Fiber 0g	Protein 37g
Total Fat 34g	Net Carbs 3g	Calories 470

% calories from

Fat 65%   Carbs 3%   Protein 31%

Herbed
Green Bean Chicken Dish

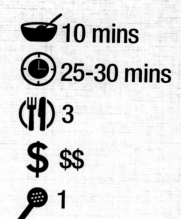

10 mins

25-30 mins

3

$ $$

1

GLUTEN FREE

DAIRY FREE

Ingredients:

- 2 whole chicken breasts
- 1 cup green beans, trimmed
- 8 cherry tomatoes, halved
- 2 Tbsp. olive oil
- 1 Tbsp. Italian seasoning
- 1 tsp. salt
- 1 tsp. black pepper

Directions:

1. Preheat a large skillet over medium heat with the olive oil.

2. Season the chicken with the Italian seasoning, salt and pepper.

3. Add the chicken to the skillet and cook for about 10 minutes each side or until cooked through.

4. Next, add the green beans and tomatoes and cook for another 5-7 minutes.

5. Enjoy right away.

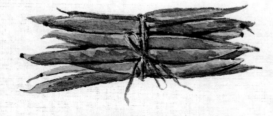

Cooking Tips:
Add four whole garlic cloves to the skillet at the same time as the green beans and tomatoes to give the dish a French twist.

Nutrition Facts (Per Serving)

Total Carbs	6g
Dietary Fiber	2g
Protein	19g
Total Fat	11g
Net Carbs	4g
Calories	196

% calories from

Fat	51%
Carbs	12%
Protein	39%

Summer
Chicken Stir Fry

🥣 10 mins

🕐 15-20 mins

🍴 4

$ $$

🔍 2

GLUTEN FREE DAIRY FREE

Ingredients:

- 4 chicken breasts, cubed
- 1 whole zucchini, sliced
- ½ cup grape tomatoes, halved
- 1 yellow onion, chopped
- 2 Tbsp. coconut oil
- 1 tsp. salt
- 1 tsp. black pepper

Directions:

1. Preheat a large skillet over medium heat with the coconut oil.

2. Add the chicken to the skillet and sauté until cooked through. This should take about 7–10 minutes.

3. Add the rest of the ingredients and sauté until the zucchini is tender.

4. Enjoy right away.

Nutrition Facts (Per Serving)

Total Carbs	5g
Dietary Fiber	1g
Protein	27g
Total Fat	10g
Net Carbs	4g
Calories	220

% calories from

Fat	41%
Carbs	9%
Protein	49%

Serving Suggestions:
Serve on top of sautéed spinach or with a side of roasted asparagus.

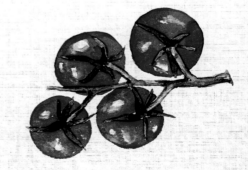

Balsamic Jumbo Shrimp

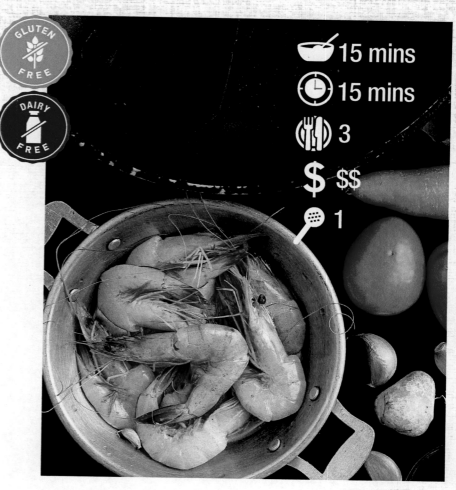

GLUTEN FREE
DAIRY FREE

🥣 15 mins
🕐 15 mins
🍴 3
$ $$
1

Ingredients:

- 12 jumbo shrimp
- 1 cup broccoli florets
- 2 cloves garlic, chopped
- 1 plum tomato, chopped
- 2 Tbsp. carrots, chopped
- 1 tsp. fresh thyme
- 3 Tbsp. balsamic vinegar
- 1 Tbsp. coconut oil
- Fresh parsley as garnish (optional)

Directions:

1. Start by heating a large skillet over medium heat with the coconut oil.

2. Add the shrimp and sauté for 5–7 minutes or until pink and cooked through.

3. Add the broccoli, garlic, tomato and carrots. Cook for another 3–4 minutes or until the vegetables are tender.

4. Add the thyme and balsamic vinegar and stir to combine.

5. Serve with a handful of parsley if desired.

Cooking Tips
Remove the tails from the shrimp before cooking if desired or keep the tails on for a fancier presentation when serving.

Serving Suggestions:
Serve with freshly ground white or black peppercorns.

Nutrition Facts (Per Serving)

Total Carbs 9g   Dietary Fiber 2g   Protein 5g   Total Fat 5g
Net Carbs 7g   Calories 101

% calories from
Fat 45%   Carbs 36%   Protein 20%

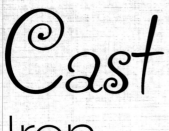

Cast Iron Braised Ribs

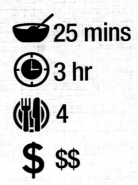
25 mins

3 hr

4

$ $$

2

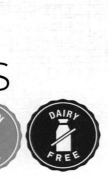

Ingredients:

- 1 lb. beef short ribs
- 2 cups reduced sodium beef broth
- 2 cloves garlic, chopped
- 1 yellow onion, chopped
- 1 carrot, chopped
- 2 Tbsp. olive oil
- 4 Tbsp. tomato paste
- 1 Tbsp. Worcestershire sauce
- 1 tsp. salt
- 1 tsp. fresh rosemary
- 1 bay leaf

Directions:

1. Start by preheating the oven to 325°F.

2. Next, season the ribs with salt and rosemary.

3. Then, heat the cast iron skillet over medium heat with the olive oil. Sear the ribs for about 10 minutes until both sides are browned.

4. While the ribs are searing, add the remaining ingredients to a mixing bowl and whisk. Add the broth to the skillet once the ribs are browned and bring the broth to a simmer.

5. Cover the skillet with the lid and allow it to cook on low for up to three hours or until super tender and cooked through.

Nutrition Facts (Per Serving)

Total Carbs 9g

Dietary Fiber 2g

Protein 17g

Total Fat 37g

Net Carbs 7g

Calories 434

% calories from

Fat 77%   Carbs 8%   Protein 16%

Cooking Tips
Check every hour to be sure that you do not need to add more broth to the skillet.

Garlic & Thyme Lamb Chops

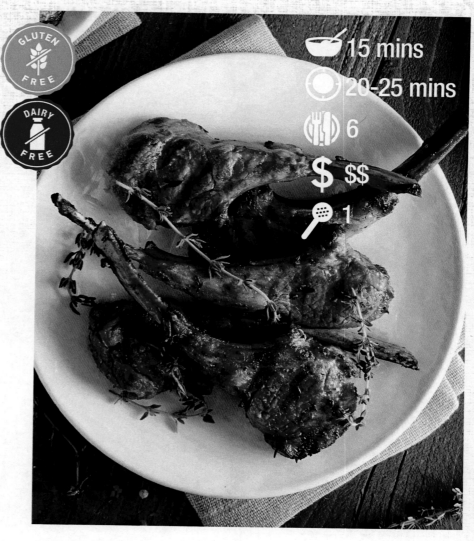

GLUTEN FREE

DAIRY FREE

🥣 15 mins

⏲ 20-25 mins

🍴 6

💲 $$

🔍 1

Ingredients:

- 6 (4 oz.) lamb chops
- 4 cloves garlic, whole
- 3 Tbsp. olive oil
- 1 tsp. ground thyme
- 2 sprigs of thyme
- 1 tsp. salt
- 1 tsp. black pepper

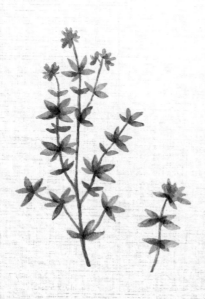

Directions:

1. Preheat a large skillet over medium heat with the olive oil.

2. Season the lamb chops with the salt, pepper and thyme.

3. Add the lamb chops to the pan with the thyme sprigs and garlic.

4. Cook about 3-4 minutes on each side.

5. Enjoy right away.

Nutrition Facts (Per Serving)

Total Carbs 1g   Dietary Fiber 0g   Protein 14g   Total Fat 21g

Net Carbs 1g   Calories 252

% calories from

Fat 75%   Carbs 2%   Protein 22%

Sesame
Fried Tofu

GLUTEN FREE

DAIRY FREE

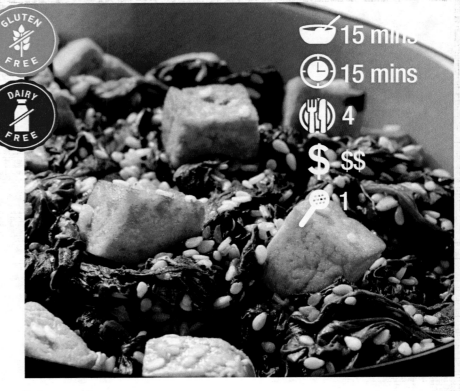

15 mins
15 mins
4
$ $$
1

Ingredients:

- 1 (14 oz.) package extra firm tofu
- 6 cups fresh spinach
- 3 cloves garlic, chopped
- ¼ cup coconut aminos
- 2 tsp. sesame oil
- 2 Tbsp. sesame seeds
- 1 Tbsp. coconut oil

Cooking Tips
If the tofu is not browning as you would like, add a teaspoon more coconut oil during cooking.

Serving Suggestions
Serve with a dash of garlic powder for a more garlicky flavor.

How to press tofu:
Drain the water from the container and move the tofu slab to a dinner plate. Place another plate on top of the tofu and top that with an object that weights 2-3 pounds, but no more than that. A large textbook works well here! Let the tofu drain for about 30 minutes before moving onto the preparation part of cooking.

Directions:

1. Remove the tofu block from the container and press (see cooking tips on how to press tofu). Next, cut the tofu into cubes.

2. Add the coconut aminos and sesame oil to a mixing bowl and add the tofu cubes. Allow the tofu to absorb the marinade for 5–10 minutes.

3. Next, preheat a large skillet over medium heat with the coconut oil. Add the tofu cubes and sauté for 7-8 minutes or until golden brown.

4. Add the garlic and spinach. Sauté for another 3-5 minutes or until the spinach is wilted.

5. Place into a large serving bowl and top with sesame seeds.

6. Split into four servings and enjoy!

Nutrition Facts (Per Serving)

Total Carbs 6g	Dietary Fiber 2g	Protein 13g	Total Fat 14g
Net Carbs 4g	Calories 188		

% calories from
Fat 62% Carbs 12% Protein 26%

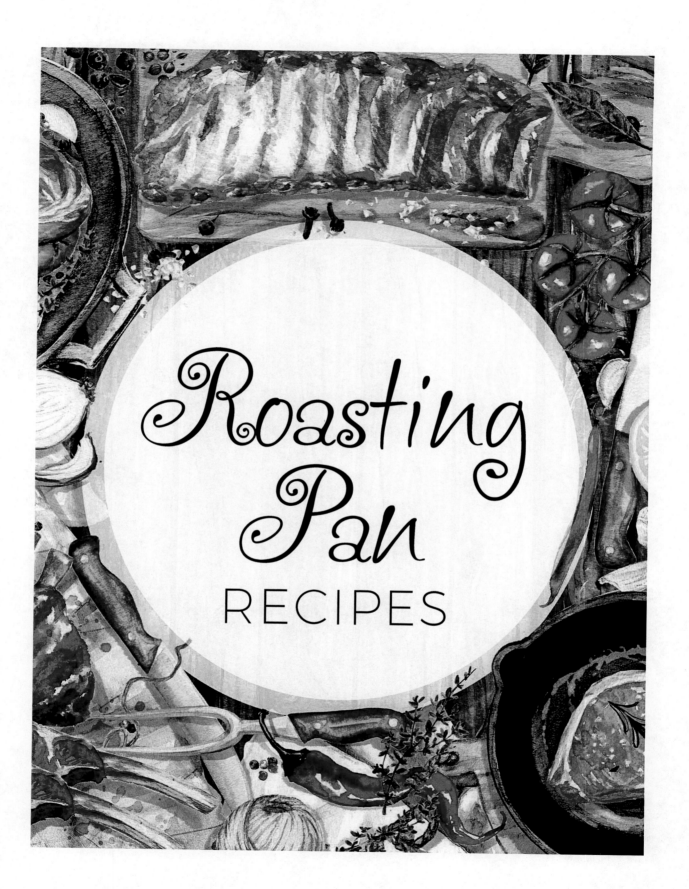

Roasting Pan
RECIPES

Spicy Beef Butternut Squash

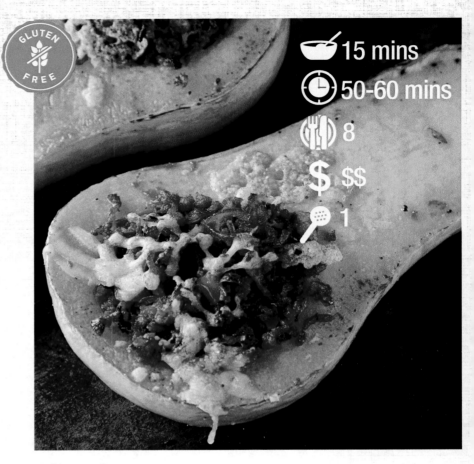

15 mins

50-60 mins

8

$$

1

Ingredients:

- 1 butternut squash
- 1 lb. ground beef, cooked
- 1 tsp. paprika
- 1 tsp. red pepper flakes
- 1 tsp. salt
- 1 tsp. black pepper
- ½ cup mozzarella cheese

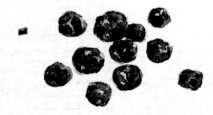

Serving Suggestions
Serve with an extra pinch of red pepper flakes to add heat if desired.

Directions:

1. Preheat the oven to 400°F and grease a roasting pan.
2. Carefully cut the butternut squash in half and remove the center and seeds. Bake for 40–45 minutes or up to a further 10 minutes until tender.
3. Next, combine the cooked ground beef and the seasonings together in a bowl.
4. Once the butternut squash is cooked, fill each squash half with half the beef mixture and top with cheese.
5. Bake for another 10–15 minutes or until the cheese starts to melt.

Nutrition Facts (Per Serving)

Total Carbs 14g   Dietary Fiber 3g   Protein 11g   Total Fat 7g
Net Carbs   11g   Calories 159

% calories from
Fat   42%   Carbs   29%   Protein   29%

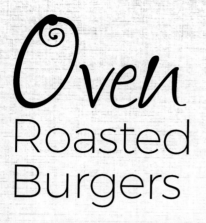

Oven
Roasted
Burgers

GLUTEN FREE

15 mins

25 mins

4

$ $$

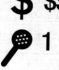
1

Ingredients:

- 1 lb. ground beef
- 1 tsp. garlic powder
- 1 tsp. onion powder
- 1 tsp. salt
- 1 tsp. black pepper
- ½ onion, thinly sliced
- 2 slices of American cheese
- 1 sliced avocado for serving (optional)

Directions:

1. Preheat the oven to 400°F and line a roasting pan with aluminum foil.
2. Add the ground beef to a large mixing bowl with the onion, garlic powder, salt and pepper. Mix to combine and form into 4 patties.
3. Place the burgers into the roasting pan and cook on one side for 10 minutes. Flip over and cook for another 10 minutes or until cooked through.
4. Add the onions and cheese and cook for 5 more minutes.
5. Serve with sliced avocado if desired.

Cooking Tips
Once the onions are added, cook until they begin to brown. If they need more than 5 minutes, increase cooking time to 10 minutes. but be careful not to burn the cheese.

Serving Suggestions
Serve with a sliced tomato if desired.

Nutrition Facts
(Per Serving)

Total Carbs	7g
Dietary Fiber	3g
Protein	19g
Total Fat	18g
Net Carbs	4g
Calories	262

% calories from

Fat	61%
Carbs	11%
Protein	29%

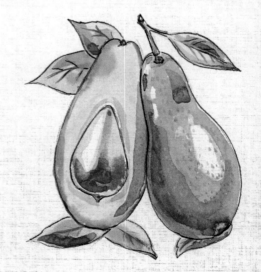

Lemon Pepper Chicken

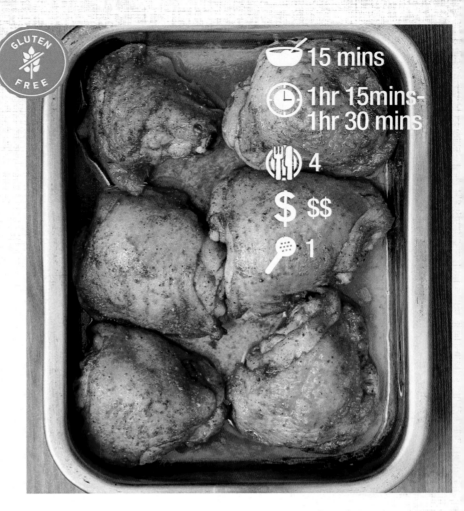

GLUTEN FREE

🥣 15 mins

🕐 1hr 15mins-1hr 30 mins

🍴 4

💲 $$

🥄 1

Ingredients:

- 4 bone-in skin-on chicken thighs
- 2 Tbsp. butter
- 2 tsp. lemon pepper seasoning
- 1 tsp. garlic powder

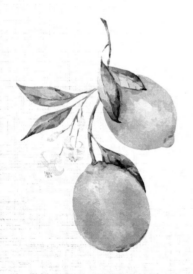

Directions:

1. Preheat the oven to 350°F and grease a roasting pan.

2. Rinse, pat the chicken thighs dry and spread the butter over the skin. Season with lemon pepper, salt and garlic powder.

3. Place the chicken thighs in the roasting pan and cover with aluminum foil. Bake for one hour at 350°F and then remove the foil and increase the temperature to 425°F. Bake for another 15–30 minutes or until the juices run clear and the thighs are brown.

Cooking Tips
Baste the chicken after one hour of cooking to prevent the chicken from drying out.

Serving Suggestions
Serve with roasted vegetables if desired.

Nutrition Facts (Per Serving)

Total Carbs 1g   Dietary Fiber 0g   Protein 15g   Total Fat 15g

Net Carbs 1g   Calories 196

% calories from

Fat 69%   Carbs 2%   Protein 31%

Oregano & Roasted Tomato Chicken

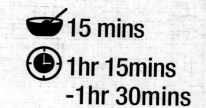

15 mins

1hr 15mins -1hr 30mins

2

$ $$

1

GLUTEN FREE   DAIRY FREE

Ingredients:

- 2 bone-in skin-on chicken legs
- 1 tsp. ground oregano
- 1 tsp. paprika
- 1 Tbsp. olive oil
- 1 Tbsp. balsamic vinegar
- 2 plum tomatoes, quartered

Directions:

1. Preheat the oven to 350°F and grease a roasting pan.

2. Rinse, pat the chicken legs dry and spread the olive oil and balsamic vinegar over the skin. Season with the oregano and paprika.

3. Place the chicken legs in the roasting pan and add the quartered tomatoes around the edges of the roasting pan. Cover with aluminum foil. Bake for one hour at 350°F and then remove the foil and increase the temperature to 425°F. Bake for another 15–30 minutes or until the juices run clear and the legs are brown.

Cooking Tips
Baste the chicken after one hour of cooking to prevent the chicken from drying out.

Serving Suggestions
Serve with a side salad.

Nutrition Facts (Per Serving)

Total Carbs	7g
Dietary Fiber	2g
Protein	16g
Total Fat	16g
Net Carbs	5g
Calories	233

% calories from

Fat	62%
Carbs	12%
Protein	27%

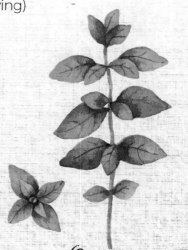

Roasted
Garlic Leg Of Lamb

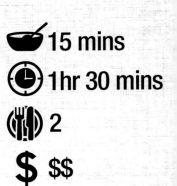

15 mins

1hr 30 mins

2

$ $$

1

GLUTEN FREE **DAIRY FREE**

Ingredients:

- 1 (2 lb.) leg of lamb
- 6 cloves garlic, chopped
- ½ cup reduced sodium beef broth
- 1 Tbsp. fresh rosemary leaves
- 2 tsp. salt
- 1 tsp. black pepper

Directions:

1. Preheat the oven to 400°F and grease a roasting pan.
2. Add the lamb to the roasting pan and pour the beef broth over the lamb and season with the garlic, rosemary leaves, salt and pepper.
3. Roast for 30 minutes and then reduce the heat to 350°F and roast for another hour or until thoroughly cooked.
4. Allow the lamb to rest for about 20 minutes before slicing.

Nutrition Facts
(Per Serving)

Total Carbs	1g
Dietary Fiber	0g
Protein	22g
Total Fat	14g
Net Carbs	1g
Calories	223

% calories from

Fat	58%
Carbs	2%
Protein	40%

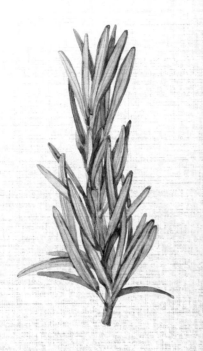

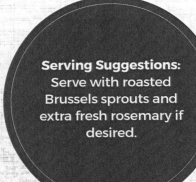

Serving Suggestions:
Serve with roasted Brussels sprouts and extra fresh rosemary if desired.

Cherry Tomato Baked Tilapia

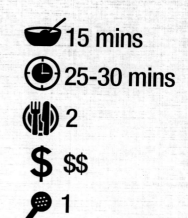

🥣 15 mins

🕐 25-30 mins

🍴 2

$ $$

🔍 1

Ingredients:

- 2 (4 oz.) tilapia fillets
- 2 tsp. butter
- ¼ cup black olives, pitted
- 8 cherry tomatoes
- ½ tsp. salt
- ¼ tsp. black pepper
- 1 tsp. garlic powder
- ¼ tsp. paprika
- 1 Tbsp. freshly squeezed lemon juice

Directions:

1. Preheat the oven to 375°F and grease a roasting pan.

2. Place the cherry tomatoes and olives in the base of the roasting pan. Add the fish fillets on top of the tomatoes.

3. Add the butter to the pan and season the fish with the salt, pepper, garlic powder, paprika and freshly squeezed lemon juice.

4. Cover the dish with aluminum foil and bake for 25–30 minutes, until the fish begins to flake easily with a fork.

Serving Suggestions
Serve with a tablespoon of balsamic vinegar if desired.

Nutrition Facts (Per Serving)

Total Carbs	6g
Dietary Fiber	2g
Protein	23g
Total Fat	8g
Net Carbs	4g
Calories	180

% calories from

Fat	38%
Carbs	13%
Protein	49%

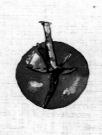 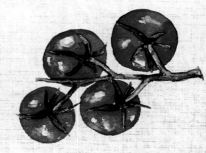

Oven Baked Zucchini Noodles With Feta

GLUTEN FREE

VEGETARIAN

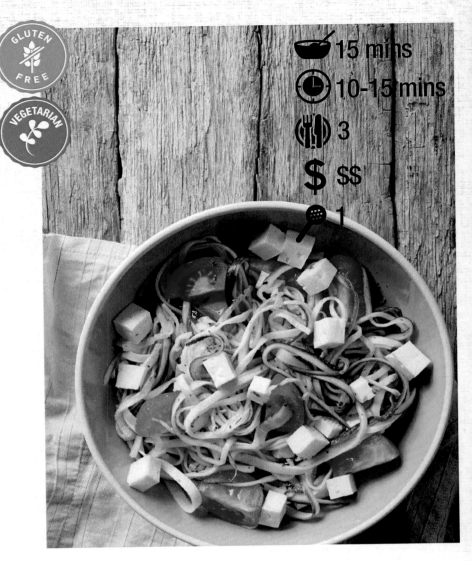

🥣 15 mins
🕐 10-15 mins
🍴 3
$ $$
🥄 1

Ingredients:

- 2 zucchini, spiralized
- 1 plum tomato, quartered
- 8 cubes feta cheese
- 1 Tbsp. olive oil
- 1 tsp. salt
- 1 tsp. black pepper

Cooking Tips:
Cook just until the zucchini is tender.

Serving Suggestions:
Serve with fresh herbs such as basil and/or thyme if desired.

Directions:

1. Preheat the oven to 375°F and grease a roasting pan.

2. Spiralize the zucchini noodles, add to the roasting pan with the olive oil and tomatoes, season with salt and pepper and bake for 10–15 minutes.

3. Next, remove from the oven and add the feta cheese cubes. Toss gently to combine and serve.

4. Enjoy right away.

Nutrition Facts (Per Serving)

Total Carbs 7g   Dietary Fiber 2g   Protein 4g   Total Fat 8g
Net Carbs 5g   Calories 105

% calories from
Fat 62%   Carbs 24%   Protein 14%

Golden Roasted Turkey

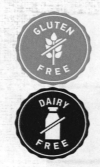
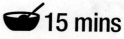

15 mins

3 hr

10

$ $$

1

Ingredients:

- 1 (10 lb.) turkey, rinsed and dried, giblets removed
- 4 Tbsp. olive oil
- 1 tsp. paprika
- 2 tsp. garlic powder
- 1 tsp. thyme
- 2 tsp. salt
- 1 tsp. pepper
- ½ cup reduced sodium chicken broth

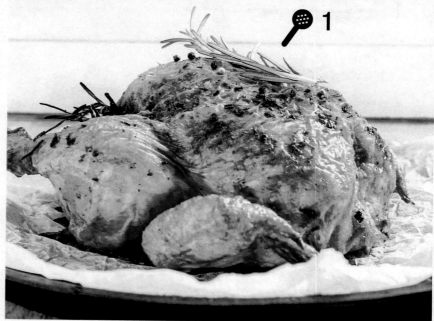

Directions:

1. Preheat the oven to 325°F and grease a roasting pan.
2. Rub the turkey with the olive oil and seasonings.
3. Add the turkey to the roasting pan, followed by the broth and roast for 3 hours or until a thermometer reads at least 165°F.
4. Allow the turkey to rest for 30 minutes before serving.

Cooking Tips:
Baste the turkey every hour during cooking to prevent it from drying out.

Serving Suggestions:
Serve with fresh herbs such as rosemary and/or thyme if desired.

Nutrition Facts (Per Serving)

Total Carbs 1g   Dietary Fiber 0g   Protein 42g   Total Fat 23g
Net Carbs 1g   Calories 391

% calories from
Fat   53%   Carbs 1%   Protein 43%

Marinara
Baked Spaghetti Squash

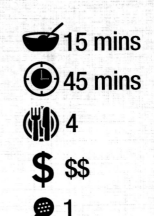

🥣 15 mins

🕐 45 mins

🍴 4

$ $$

🥄 1

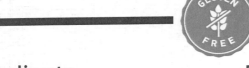

Ingredients:

- 1 spaghetti squash
- ½ cup no sugar added marinara sauce
- ½ cup mushrooms, sliced
- 1 Tbsp. olive oil
- 1 tsp. salt
- 1 tsp. black pepper
- ¼ cup shredded mozzarella cheese

Directions:

1. Preheat the oven to 375°F and grease a roasting pan.

2. Carefully cut the spaghetti squash in half and remove the center and seeds. Season with salt, pepper and olive oil and flip upside down on the pan. Bake for 35 minutes or until the squash is easily removed with a fork, adding 10 minutes of extra cooking time if needed.

3. Next, add the mushrooms and marinara sauce to the cavities of the squash and top with the shredded cheese. Bake for another 10 minutes.

4. Enjoy right away.

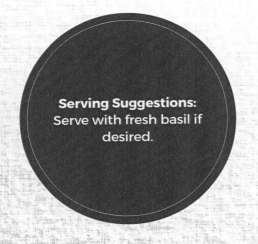

Serving Suggestions:
Serve with fresh basil if desired.

Nutrition Facts (Per Serving)

Total Carbs	9g
Dietary Fiber	2g
Protein	3g
Total Fat	6g
Net Carbs	7g
Calories	92

% calories from

Fat	59%
Carbs	39%
Protein	13%

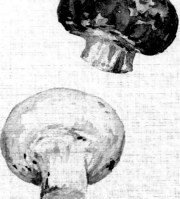

Lemon
Roasted
Vegetables

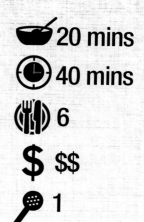

🥣 20 mins
🕐 40 mins
🍴 6
$ $$
🥄 1

GLUTEN FREE · DAIRY FREE · VEGETARIAN

Ingredients:

- 2 zucchini, sliced
- 1 cup button mushrooms
- 8 large grape tomatoes
- 10 asparagus spears, chopped
- 1 yellow pepper, chopped
- 1 Tbsp. freshly squeezed lemon juice
- 2 Tbsp. olive oil
- ½ tsp. salt

Directions:

1. Preheat the oven to 450°F.

2. Chop and slice the vegetables according to the ingredients list above and place them in an oiled roasting pan.

3. Toss with the lemon juice and olive oil and season with salt.

4. Roast for 40 minutes, stirring every 10 minutes.

Nutrition Facts (Per Serving)

Total Carbs	5g
Dietary Fiber	2g
Protein	2g
Total Fat	5g
Net Carbs	3g
Calories	65

% calories from

Fat	62%
Carbs	27%
Protein	11%

Cooking Tips:
If the vegetables are getting too brown too quickly, reduce the heat to 425°F.

Serving Suggestions:
Serve with lemon zest if desired.

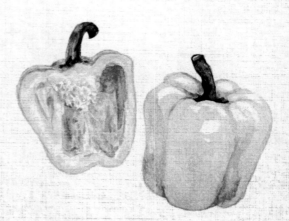

My Favorite Pots & Pans

Below are my favorite pots and pans that I use in the kitchen. You may already have your favorite, but if you are looking for some recommendations then the below might help.

Slow Cooker

- Crock-Pot SCCPVL610-S 6-Quart Programmable Cook and Carry Oval Slow Cooker, Digital Timer, Stainless Steel:I love this stainless-steel crockpot as it's very practical, affordable, and holds six quarts. You can also choose a wide variety of cooking times from 30 minutes up to 20 hours, making it very versatile. The best part is how easy it is to clean, which makes slow cooking even easier!

  On Amazon - http://geni.us/scooker

Skillets

- T-fal E91898 Ultimate Hard Anodized Scratch Resistant Titanium Nonstick Thermo-Spot Heat Indicator Anti-Warp Base Dishwasher Safe Oven Safe PFOA Free Glass Lid Cookware, 12-Inch, Gray: This is one of my favorite skillets to use as it's scratch resistant, non-stick, oven safe, and dishwasher safe. It's basically an all in one product, so I use this for just about any recipe I need a skillet for. I also find this skillet to be super durable and convenient to use when transferring back and forth from the stove to the oven or the stove to the sink as this skillet comes with silicone sleeves. The best part about this skillet is that is comes with Thermo-Spot Technology to indicate when the pan is ready! How great is that! No more guessing if your pan is heated enough to start cooking. For the cost, you really can't beat a pan like this.

  On Amazon - http://geni.us/pans

- Cuisinart 722-22 Chef's Classic Stainless 9-Inch Open Skillet: This is my favorite stainless steel skillet. I find that the pan heats up very quickly and I also love the fact that the pan is built with a rim to help prevent your food from spilling over when you transfer your food to a plate. This particular product also comes in a few different pan sizes so you can buy one for your individual cooking needs.

  On Amazon - http://geni.us/Skillet

Roasting Pans

- Calphalon Contemporary Hard Anodized Nonstick 16-Inch Roasting Pan with Rack 5 pc. Set: This is my favorite nonstick roasting pan that comes with some other add-on features as well. It comes with a rack to make cooking whole chickens and turkeys so much easier. I also find this pan to be pretty easy to carry as not all roasting pans are easy to transport between the oven and the counter top, especially when hot! This is an awesome set that will last many years and works well for so many recipes.

  On Amazon - http://geni.us/roasting

- Cuisinart Chef's Classic Stainless 16-Inch Rectangular Roaster with Rack: If you prefer a stainless-steel rather than a nonstick roasting pan, this is a beautifully made stainless steel roasting pan. This pan was designed for drip-free pouring, and although it's very sturdy, it's also pretty lightweight which is a huge plus.

  On Amazon - http://geni.us/roasting2

Instant Pot

- Instant Pot IP-DUO60 7-in-1 Multi-Functional Pressure Cooker, 6Qt/1000W: These instant pots are becoming increasingly popular, and that's because they make cooking so much easier and less time-consuming! I love this instant pot because it serves as a 7-in-1 multifunctional cooker. You can use it as a pressure cooker, slow cooker, and steamer just to name a few. I also find that I get really great results when cooking with this as it seems to tenderize meats extremely well and steams vegetables to perfection! This is definitely something worth investing in if you want a product that does it all.

  On Amazon - http://geni.us/instantpot1

You May Also Like

Please visit the below link for other books by the author

http://geni.us/ElizJane

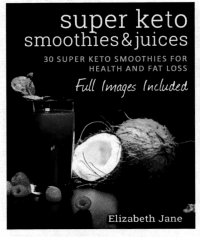

super keto smoothies & juices
30 SUPER KETO SMOOTHIES FOR HEALTH AND FAT LOSS
Full Images Included
Elizabeth Jane

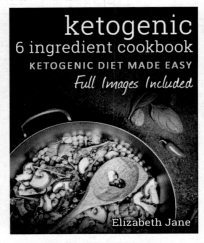

ketogenic 6 ingredient cookbook
KETOGENIC DIET MADE EASY
Full Images Included
Elizabeth Jane

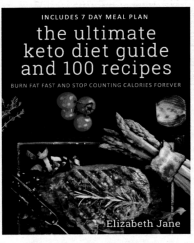

INCLUDES 7 DAY MEAL PLAN
the ultimate keto diet guide and 100 recipes
BURN FAT FAST AND STOP COUNTING CALORIES FOREVER
Elizabeth Jane

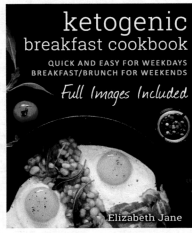

ketogenic breakfast cookbook
QUICK AND EASY FOR WEEKDAYS BREAKFAST/BRUNCH FOR WEEKENDS
Full Images Included
Elizabeth Jane

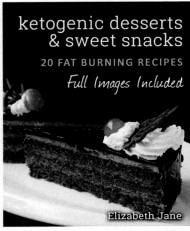

ketogenic desserts & sweet snacks
20 FAT BURNING RECIPES
Full Images Included
Elizabeth Jane

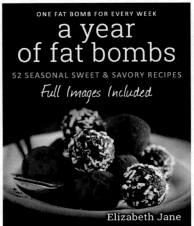

ONE FAT BOMB FOR EVERY WEEK
a year of fat bombs
52 SEASONAL SWEET & SAVORY RECIPES
Full Images Included
Elizabeth Jane

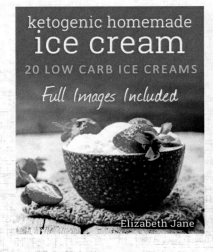

ketogenic homemade ice cream
20 LOW CARB ICE CREAMS
Full Images Included
Elizabeth Jane

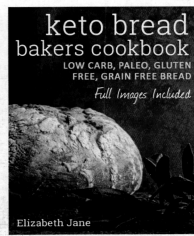

keto bread bakers cookbook
LOW CARB, PALEO, GLUTEN FREE, GRAIN FREE BREAD
Full Images Included
Elizabeth Jane

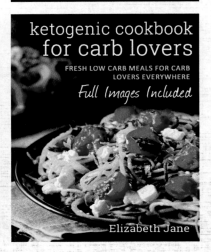

ketogenic cookbook for carb lovers
FRESH LOW CARB MEALS FOR CARB LOVERS EVERYWHERE
Full Images Included
Elizabeth Jane

50460516R00043